Forever Young

by

Earlyne Chaney, Ph.D.

Astara's Library of
Body/Mind/Spirit Masterworks

Published by

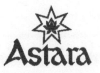

Astara

800 W. Arrow Highway
Upland, CA 91786

First Edition, 1990

Cover design: Teodors A. Liliensteins
Photo Model: Nancey J. Harrison

Copyright © 1990 by Astara, Inc.
Library of Congress Catalogue Card Number 90-84224
ISBN 0-918936-22-5

Printed in the United States of America

DEDICATION

This book is lovingly dedicated to Grace Cooper, my devoted secretary, without whose love and steadfast service the work I have completed during the latter years of my life would not have been possible. Our organization manual calls her my "secretary," but I call her my companion, my co-worker, my dearest friend and my sister soul. My gratitude is without measure, since Earth's measurements could never compute the depths and reach of my heart's love.

Other books by Earlyne Chaney

Remembering — The Autobiography of a Mystic
The Masters and Astara
Secrets From Mount Shasta
The Book of Beginning Again
Revelations of Things to Come
Beyond Tomorrow — a Book of Prophecies
Shining Moments of a Mystic
Initiation in the Great Pyramid
(published by Astara, Inc.)

- - - - - - - - - - -

The Mystery of Death and Dying
(Initiation at the Moment of Death)
The Eyes Have It
(published by Samuel Weiser, Inc.)

- - - - - - - - - - -

Astara's Book of Life
(A series of esoteric teachings of the
Mystery Schools of all ages)

- - - - - - - - - - -

Books in Collaboration
Kundalini and the Third Eye
(With William Messick)
The Mystical Marriage of Science and Spirit
By Frances Paelian
(Based on the teachings of Earlyne Chaney)

A MESSAGE FROM ASTARA

The publishers of this book have made it available to you in the belief that it will make a contribution to your life on its various important levels: physical, emotional, intellectual, and spiritual.

Actually, we consider this volume to be an extension of the teachings contained in Astara's series of mystical studies known as *Astara's Book of Life*. The lessons comprising the *Book of Life* are distributed on a world-wide basis only to members of Astara. Astara was founded in 1951 as a non-profit religious organization including the following concepts:

1. A center of all religions, oriented to mystical Christianity but accepting and teaching all religions as beneficial to humankind.

2. A school of the ancient Mysteries, offering a compendium of the esoteric teachings of all ages.

3. A fraternity of all philosophies, coordinating many viewpoints of humankind and the interacting inner structures which unite us as one in the infinite.

4. An institute of psychic research, with emphasis on spiritual healing of physical, emotional and mental aspects, and to life before and after physical incarnation.

If these areas of interest are appealing to you, you may wish to pursue the studies of *Astara's Book of Life* as have thousands of others in some ninety countries around the world.

To give you information about Astara, its teachings, and other possible services to you, we have prepared a treatise entitled *Finding Your Place in the Golden Age*. You may have it without cost or obligation. Write:

Astara
P.O. Box 5003
Upland, CA 91786-5003

ACKNOWLEDGMENTS

My first debt of gratitude goes to my devoted and dedicated "computer secretary," Phyllis Harrison, whose skill at her keyboard made this book possible — and to her assistant, Fran Blaye. Next, to my husband, Robert, and his secretary, Shirley Pearson, whose editing rounded out my square writings. The long hours each of these co-workers spent in rewriting and polishing cannot be measured in monetary computations, but only in measurements of the heart. And these can only be equated by a Higher Source, in whose Book of Life the work of their hands is surely recorded and will be rewarded.

Chapter Four
Healing Skin Problems 59

A NOTE FROM THE PUBLISHER

The products, remedies, formulas and ideas in this book are not in any way offered as medical advice or prescriptions for the relief or cure of any illness whatsoever. Nor is any diagnosis intended or implied.

Neither author nor publisher intends that the contents of this book replace competent medical advice given by a duly authorized professional. The book reflects the author's personal research and experience which may or may not parallel those of the reader.

Any company's products are more, or less, effective for one person than those of another company. In the final analysis, each person needs to experiment and compare for himself or herself to judge results personally.

Neither author nor publisher receives payment for any product listed or recommended in this book. Inclusion of products and companies was entirely at the discretion of the author and based upon her personal experiences and research.

Introduction

This book is about "looking good" as one of the mystical aspects of staying young — and even to roll back the onslaught of age! It's a spin-off from *The You Book: A Treasury of Health and Healing* which I wrote to cover many facets of health and well-being. When I first began the *The You Book* manuscript, I felt that maintaining youth would be as important as health, which is the central theme of the writings. But many of my readers sent an avalanche of health ideas to be published in the book, so much so that the writings became voluminous.

It became obvious the youth aspect must be deleted to form a separate publication, or much of the health information must be omitted — which was unthinkable. So two books were created. *The You Book* is a companion to this one, but each is a separate entity. Youth and beauty go hand in hand with health and well-being. There's an old adage which says, "When you look good, you feel good."

It's hoped that, following the premise of these writings, you'll look so good, health and well-being will be a natural happening. And while you're getting healthy, handsome and happy, don't forget to add holy, the spiritual aspect:

Healthy, Handsome, Happy, Holy

No better words to live by.

Earlyne Chaney, Ph.D.

Chapter One

First --
the Face

In *The Book of Beginning Again* I told the story of Sanford Bennett. Ill and discouraged at age 54, he restored his health and his body to a remarkable degree through exercises now recognized as isometrics: tensing and releasing muscles. Photographs of Bennett in a book he published, long out of print, demonstrated many isometrics which transformed not only his body but his facial muscles. The techniques which restored his body were reprinted in *The Book of Beginning Again* .* But in that

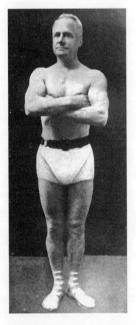

Sanford Bennett age 72

*At your bookstore or order from Astara, Box 5003 , Upland, CA 91785-5003

book I did not speak at length concerning his facial techniques, preferring to present them in this particular publication. The facial techniques Bennett presented in his book were obviously beneficial to and for him. His photographs clearly indicate that he was able to restore his

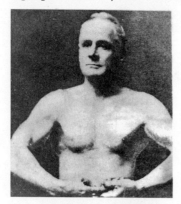

Sanford Bennett

face to that of a man much younger than his 72 years. His facial muscles were firm, strong, free of wrinkles and other signs of aging.

The facial techniques he offers require facial massage. For him they obviously were extremely successful. He suggests contracting the muscles, then stroking upward to firm the underlying muscles. Yet, as in all things, there is a controversy. In discussing his facial massage with others, some have suggested his method may stretch the skin, possibly resulting in wrinkles. As for myself, I have used his massage techniques for years and have found them extremely effective. They are offered for your consideration but I also present my own techniques, developed over long periods of trial, leaving you, the reader, to make the choice. I use not only his facial massage but also exercises which tighten muscles. The first part of this chapter contains the teachings and techniques offered by Sanford Bennett, the second half are mine. Study them well and select your own preferences. Or perhaps, like me, you'll choose both.

(Throughout the book you'll find products suggested that have been found conducive to youth and beauty. I've used many of them myself so can "testify" to their effectiveness. I am forever seeking those that are "natural," that is, containing little or no harmful or toxic chemicals. These seem to qualify. Those that have been selected are: Fanie International, [pronounced Fanay]; Beleza Beauty Products; Patricia Allison Products; Creative Illusions Natural Cosmetics [holistically formulated]. Others are mentioned briefly but these will be mentioned over and over. In the last chapter, you'll find full information about the individual products, their ingredients, their distributors, and where they may be ordered. So when you read, "address elsewhere," seek for it in the last chapter.)

The following are Bennett's own words concerning his facial techniques, taken from his book:

Rejuvenation of the Face, Throat, and Neck (via Sanford Bennett)

"The exercises I have described, if persistently and methodically practiced, will surely restore to an aged body much of the lost strength and elasticity of an earlier period of life.* For it is possible in this way to restore to the muscles of age the rounded contour they once possessed. But if the muscles of the face and neck are neglected, they will present the relaxed and flabby condition characteristic of old age even though the rest of the body has been developed to the strength of an athlete. Unless the facial muscles are also exercised, the face and the neck may show the wear and deterioration of years in marked contrast to the apparently more youthful body.

"If you exercise those muscles just as you exercise the muscles of the body, they will surely grow in size, strength

*See *The Book of Beginning Again*

and elasticity. The hollow places in the neck and cheeks will fill up. The muscles which surround the eyes can be increased in plumpness and, with a treatment I will now describe, that smoothness of skin, characteristic of youth may, to a very considerable extent, be regained. And this much-to-be-desired condition can be accomplished without cost. If a face ointment is desired during the friction, use pure olive oil or any good natural face cream or moisturizer."

(Note from Earlyne — Be careful of your choice of oils and creams. Many contain rancid oils and harmful chemicals and dyes not only perilous to your facial skin but your entire health. Read the labels. You may want to use any of Fanie's night creams or oils, which will *not* be rancid because they are fractured and stabilized with PCMX. Or a product called Beleza which contains honey. Both contain all the good vitamins and minerals. The honey of Beleza forms a good base to massage the face and throat muscles with upward strokes while still lying in bed, after you awaken. It's better for those with dry skin. Or you may want to order Patricia Allison's Massage Oil which contains safflower oil, apricot kernel oil, sweet almond oil and a multitude of vitamins. In the last chapter you'll read more about all these products and where to order. You may prefer a good Aromatherapy Oil. Or mix your own sesame, olive, wheat germ and avocado. The avocado oil is pure protein. All such oils, including the olive oil suggested by Bennett, should be cold pressed.)

"The moisturizer will soften the outer skin and, after being rubbed in, will leave it cleaner, clearer and soft. But the true secret of restoring the smoothness of youth is friction. The skin can be polished and the wrinkles rubbed out like any other piece of leather, and the palms of the hands and the tips of the fingers are the very best tools to use for that purpose. This polishing, wrinkle-removing process can best be done while you lie comfortably in bed, as in that position it is easier, it is less fatiguing, and you can get at the wrinkles more readily lying down than when either sitting or standing.

"We know that living tissue can only be formed by the digestive process. Thus it is folly to believe the skin can be fully nourished only by applying exterior oils or creams. They are a valuable aid, to be sure — but skin, to be beautiful, must also be nourished from within through foods and liquids. If by only rubbing skin cream into the skin it was possible to 'plump up' one's cheeks, throat and chin and, in that way, generally make oneself beautiful, a kind of physical millennium would ensue. All elderly and wrinkled people would soon become attractively young. Application of exterior creams alone simply will not accomplish such a miracle. But the proper pure natural oils *plus* friction massage *plus* pure natural foods *will* restore and rejuvenate the face. Persistent friction of the skin, and plenty of it, using the palms of the hands and tips of the fingers will accomplish miracles. The moisturizer will act as a lubricant in preventing the skin from becoming chafed in the rubbing process.

"The usual objection made to the friction process I advise is that the skin might loosen and the pores might become enlarged. If you go at it too vigorously on a dry skin, that is very possible. But if care is taken it will not happen. And, even if it did, as soon as the minute muscles and structure of the skin tone up under the stimulating treatment, that condition will speedily disappear and improvement will surely result. So don't go at this method of facial rejuvenation too energetically. If you do you will get sore and discouraged. The same rule applies to massaging the face and throat as to any other system of exercise. Go slow, stick to it, and you will succeed. The following are my methods:

"While still lying in bed, cup the chin upon the palms of the hands. Tense the throat muscles. Press firmly and rub the muscle under the chin with vigorous upward strokes. Include the entire throat, alternating the hands. Stroke from the base of the throat upward, continually shifting. Be sure to tense the throat muscles.

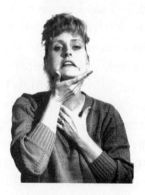

Tense the throat muscles

"The jaws are covered by broad flat muscular bands commencing underneath the jawbone and running upward toward the cheekbones to which they are attached. These jaw muscles readily respond and can be developed by deep massage. This should be practiced along the edge of the jawbone using the heel of the hand. Deep firm rubbing of the muscles of the jaws while the jaws are tensed will develop these muscles. This treatment will speedily tone up and increase the size of these muscles, thus giving a rounded and more youthful appearance to the lines of the jaw.

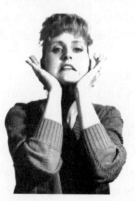

Deep firm rubbing

"As years creep on, the cheeks sink in and hollows

appear where once they were full and plump. This is due to the shrinking of the supporting muscles. These are voluntary muscles and can be exercised at will just as you can exercise the muscles of the arms and legs. And, just as exercise of any part of the body will improve it, so exercise of the muscles of the face will have the same effect. As with the (isometric) body exercises, I practice these facial exercises before rising in the morning.

"1. Draw up both corners of the mouth toward the eyes, or in the position of an exaggerated smile. This will bunch up those supporting muscles on the upper part of the cheek bones, and immediately below the corners of the eyes.

"2. Now drop the chin to its utmost extent. This will place a further tension upon the cheek supporting muscles.

"3. In this position — that is, keeping them bunched up — alternately open and close the jaws, at the same time steadily massage, or rub, with the palms of the hands, using firm upward strokes."
(Note from Earlyne: — Begin at the base of the throat. Stroke upward over the entire throat, jaw line, cheeks, temples, and forehead. If the night cream applied at bedtime the night before needs replenishing, apply a pat or two. If you've chosen Beleza, its honey base makes it 'tacky' on the skin, and the massage removes the outer dead cells. The mas-

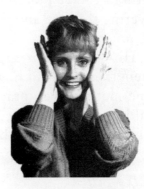

Stroke upward

sage brings fresh blood to the area. Be sure to keep muscles tensed.) "This will infallibly enlarge them, for the logical reasons described. The result will be that the overlying skin and tissue, being well supported, will give to the cheeks the rounded appearance of earlier years. There will also be an increase in color and a generally improved and more youthful appearance. This exercise will not produce any lines upon your face, and will certainly develop the supporting muscles of your cheeks.

"Rejuvenation of the face and throat is principally dependent upon your success in developing the muscles which underlie and support the skin and other covering tissue. For if the supporting muscles are weak, loose and shrunken, then no matter how brilliant the complexion may be, a youthful appearance is impossible, and any artificial coloring only emphasizes any 'saggy' indications of age. If those muscles can be developed and strengthened to support the underlying structure, as they did in earlier years, then a more youthful appearance will surely result. This is written for both sexes, and briefly describes the methods I have practiced for the improvement of the skin covering the face and throat, also the underlying supporting muscles.

"How then can sagging muscles be toned up and strengthened? And how can hollows be built up? By the same methods you practice when you are endeavoring to build up your arms, legs, or any other part of your body. Muscular activity — that is, exercise — is the secret. For all muscles have this property: when they are *not* exercised they will shrink, thus losing their elasticity. Then the marks that we know as the indications of age will appear.

"Alternately contracting and relaxing the muscles of the arms and legs will make them increase in size, strength and elasticity, and exactly the same thing occurs when you persistently and systematically contract and massage — that is, rub firmly — any muscle of the face. The skin, like any other piece of leather, is improved by friction, and the very best instruments for polishing it up are the palms and fingers. Also this friction process will remove the fine superficial lines which commence to appear with the advancing years, when the texture of the skin is therefore not as fine as formerly.

"This can be accomplished by contracting and bunching up the cheek muscles. Then press firmly with the palm of the hand upon the cheek you commence with. And rub those bunched muscles firmly, deliberately and well towards the temples or corners of the eyes. Ten or fifteen upward movements will be sufficient to commence, but gradually increase every morning until you have determined the length of time advisable in your case. After massaging one cheek, repeat upon the other, or, if you prefer, massage both at once. This exercise will strengthen the large circular muscle which surrounds the eye and, when developed, will prevent sagginess there. It will also strengthen and develop the cheek muscles and, when this is done, the hollows will disappear.

"The mouth is encircled by a wide muscular band. As we advance in years, if that muscle is not exercised it will atrophy and become weaker, the mouth will sag and droop at the corners. Deep lines will extend from those points downward, the result being the slack mouth of age. My mouth does not droop at the corners, but is as firm and muscular as it was when I was 50 years younger. This is due to an exercise I practice for strengthening the sphincter muscle encircling the mouth.

"I insert my little fingers in the corners of my mouth.

Then I alternately tense the lips, pull and relax. I pull the

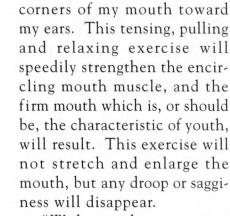

corners of my mouth toward my ears. This tensing, pulling and relaxing exercise will speedily strengthen the encircling mouth muscle, and the firm mouth which is, or should be, the characteristic of youth, will result. This exercise will not stretch and enlarge the mouth, but any droop or sagginess will disappear.

Tense, pull, relax

"With age, the supporting muscles of the temple usually sink, and the sunken temples of age appear. They should be developed and filled up by exercise, that is, persistent firm rubbing of these temple muscles, which will remedy this trouble. And frequent friction of the temple should begin well toward the corners of the eyes, using the heel of the hand in an upward outward movement

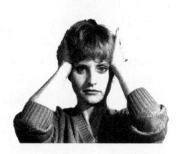

Upward, outward

toward the temple. It will produce the smooth temples of youth, and also will remove crow's feet."

****

This concludes Sanford Bennett's facial massage. I have practiced this upward massage, upon awakening, for years to great benefit. I use *Beleza's Anti-Aging Cream* or *Fanie's Mist-E-Oil*, but you should use an oil of your choice.

Facial Exercises

After reading the Bennett book and observing the incredible results of his exercises in bed, I began not only the practice of his isometric techniques for the body, but also the facial massages at the same time. Consider ending your body exercises with the one suggesting that a pillow be placed beneath the shoulders while lying on the back. After raising and lowering the head several times, allow the head to remain tilted back, the chin pointed toward the ceiling. Try touching your nose with your bottom lip, tensing every muscle of the face and throat and holding to the count of twelve. Then move the tensing action to the left and then the right so that the muscles 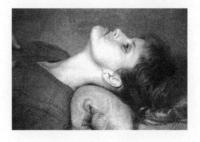 of the sides of the throat are exercised, always holding, tensing then relaxing. While the chin is tilted back and the throat muscles tensed, place your palms under your chin as Bennett suggests and apply upward strokes. After completing this exercise, replace the pillow under your head and continue with the facial exercises. The facial exercises require lying on the back. All are extremely effective. You may combine these with Bennett's facial massage, as I do. These are my choices:

Tense and relax

1. To firm the muscles in the lower face, especially around the mouth and cheeks, first relax the face. Slowly form an "O" with the lips, projecting the lips forward. Now slowly pull the lips backward, tensing the lips, cheeks and throat as you smile an exaggerated smile, contracting

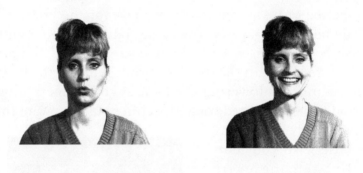

"O"   Exercise # 1   Smile!

the muscles strongly and hold. Repeat several times, projecting the lips, contracting in a hard firm smile, tensing. Then relax.

2. Now move the lips to the right, pulling the corners downward. Tense and hold to the count of twelve. Now repeat with the corners of the lips moved to the left and downward. Again tense and hold to the count of twelve. Now turn the corner of the lips upward toward the right eye, tense and hold. Then toward the left eye, tensing and holding. Now raise the right corner of the upper lip and tense in a scowl. Tense every muscle of the face and throat and hold to twelve. Repeat on the left side.

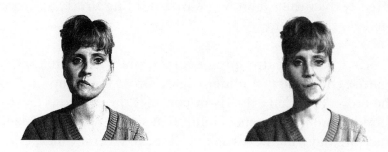

Exercise # 2   Tense and hold

3. For firming the eye muscles and removing "crow's feet," first relax the face. Now place the tip of the third finger on the bone at the outer corners of the eyes. Gently contract your eyes, cheeks and temples, not simply the muscles under the eyes. Hold the contraction for a count of six, then release the tension and open slowly. Repeat the contraction-releasing several times slowly, never rapidly. It is an isometric exercise and the secret of success is to tense and hold, tense and hold. Be sure the pad of the fingertip rests ever so lightly at the corner of each eye and only tighten the pressure while squeezing the eyes. If you tighten the pressure of the fingers and pull outward it will stretch the skin. Also, while massaging with the hands, as Bennett has suggested, use the heel of the hands to stroke upward from the corner of each eye toward the temples.

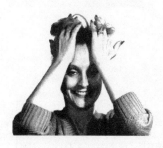

Exercise # 3

An alternate technique: Place the heels of the hands directly over the eyebrows. While holding firmly, squeeze the eyes downward.

4. To correct drooping eyelids, place the fingertips against the bone just under the eyebrows. Look upward to the brows to widen eyes. Now contract the eyebrows downward toward the fingers. Hold, then slowly release the contraction and widen eyes again. Repeat several times, contracting, holding and releasing very slowly. Try to avoid frowning. Concentrate on the eyelids and avoid contracting the lines between the eyebrows.

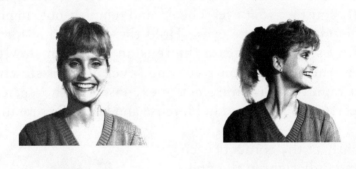

Center   Exercise # 5   Left

5. For throat and neck rejuvenation, contract the lips in a wide hard smile and turn head, first to the left then back to the center and release. Contract again and turn the face to the right, back to the center and release. Repeat several times.

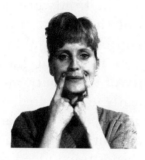

6. For lines around lips, place forefingers on the corners of the lips. Hold while contracting the lips. That is, pull back with fingers while contracting the lips forward in a whistling motion.

Exercise # 6

7. Form mouth into an "O." Next suck in the cheeks. The jaw will automatically drop. Hold the tension for a count of six. Repeat this exercise several times. It firms the entire face.

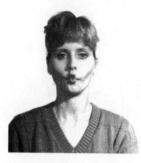

Exercise # 7

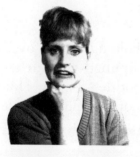

Exercise # 8

8. To firm the chin line, rest your chin on a fist. Open your mouth wide against resistance from the fist. Hold the tension. Close slowly, still tensing jaw and throat muscles. Repeat several times.

9. Nothing so clearly discloses inner tension as the tight clenched muscles of the jaw or the firmly gripped muscles of the lips — taut, tight strictures that hold the mouth too firm and hard. Flexibility of the mouth muscles is greatly to be desired, not only for inner poise, peace and relaxation, but for beauty and a happy disposition. Open the mouth slightly and turn the tongue upward to the roof of the palate. Rub gently with the tip of the tongue, tensing the muscles of the lower face and throat.

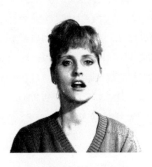

Exercise # 9

Practice a back and forth movement, tensing as the tongue moves forward to the back of the teeth. Then relax the tongue. Repeat this movement several times.

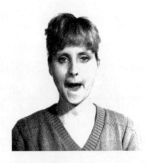

10. Folding the lips over the teeth, open the mouth in a wide "toothless" smile. Hold to a count of six. Slowly release the tension, then repeat.

Exercise # 10

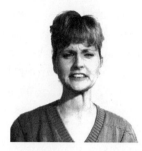 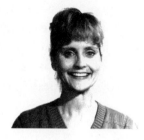

Exercise
11

A, E, I, O, U

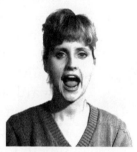

(See page
18 for
details.)

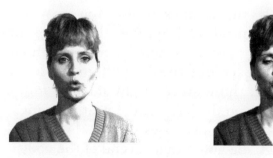

11. Say the vowels A-E-I-O-U. But exaggerate with wide firm mouth movements — that is, A with the tensed mouth open and wide, E with the teeth and jaws clenched together in a wide exaggerated smile, I with the mouth opened wide and the eyebrows raised in surprise, O by making an O of the lips and tensing all the muscles around the lips, U (oo) by pursing the contracted lip and throat muscles.

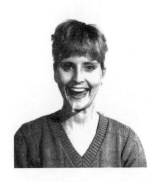

Exercise # 12

12. To destroy a double chin or a fat pouch under the chin, t ry this: say *"cat"* greatly exaggerating all the facial muscles. Tense every muscle of the face and neck. Touch under the chin to discover how the muscle under the chin is drawn inward and upward. If you have time for only one facial exercise, choose this one. It is superb for the entire face and neck.

This concludes the facial exercises. You are now ready to turn on your right side and continue the body exercises. If you have a busy morning schedule, you may choose to practice the body exercises thusly: perform those on the back one morning, those on the right side the following morning, and those on the left side the next morning. But the facial massage and exercises should always be done lying on the back. Be aware that several of the body exercises contribute to strengthening the facial and throat muscles. As both body and facial exercises are continued,

it is my firm conviction that you will see a new you gradually emerging. Certainly the contours of the physical
form will firm and become more symmetrical. Simultaneously, as the muscles all over the body are contracted and
relaxed, all the toxins in the body begin to flow into the
bloodstream and the organs of elimination, purifying the
system. As the encrusted deposits of the arteries, the uric
acids in the muscles, and the toxins in the bloodstream
begin to depart the body, so does the new you begin to experience a rejuvenation, an amazing insurge of energy, a
spark of renewed life force, a balanced flow of the positive-
negative pranic force throughout your total being.

As the physical is purified, so do the channels of spiritual receptivity respond. The auric forcefield of the new
You-niverse begins to indraw a higher cosmic substance
and you experience a total rebirth — physically, mentally,
psychically and spiritually. Again, for the rejuvenation
of the muscles of the body see *The Book of Beginning Again*.

Chapter Two

Next -- the Skin

Cleansing the Skin

Totally apart from their facial youth aspect, there is much to be said concerning the skin. But since in this present writing we are focusing on facial youth, and retaining it, nothing is more important than keeping the skin clean. A man has little difficulty in cleansing his face — he simply splashes it with soap and water, rinses it and pats it dry with a towel. Too frequently he splashes it with some highly advertised aftershave, which usually is totally detrimental. The male, however, is rapidly becoming aware of the wisdom of applying a moisturizing lotion after shaving. But his cleansing process usually focuses on soap and water.

On the other hand, a woman faces a decision, a most controversial decision — whether to soap or to cleanse with cream. The entire cosmetic industry is divided in this controversy. Some strongly advocate soap while the other camp stoutly insists on creams and lotions. Personally, I never use bar soap. I prefer liquid cleansers because bar soap requires a solidifying agent such as wax which leaves a film on the skin so that the moisturizer cannot penetrate and perform its necessary function. Bar soaps coat the skin with calcium and soap scum.

If you must use a bar soap, seek for milder soaps in health stores. Check your labels for the best possible choice for your particular skin type. Facial soaps rich in oils and fats are good choices for dry or normal skins because their fat content may prevent thorough removal of all oil from the skin. Not a good choice for those with oily skin. Those with very dry or irritated skin may wish to select French Milled soap, which contains very little alkalinity. This will help the skin retain some measure of its natural acid mantle. Avoid all detergent soaps for both the face and the bath as they are extremely harsh and irritating. Always choose soft soaps, hopefully devoid of some of the objectionable solidifying waxes. Most health store soaps will contain herbs, oils, oatmeal and other natural cleansers with fewer harsh chemicals. Avoid those containing fragrances.

Instead of bar soaps, consider liquid cleansers with plant derivatives. Fanie offers two forms from white oak bark. One comes in a brown liquid, the other in a white liquid cream which looks like thick milk. They are made totally of natural herbs and plants. Chemical free. They were formulated by a renowned chemist, the late Clyde Johnson, and marketed by his wife Florence under the name of Fanie Products. *Fanie's White Oak*

Bark Cleanser contains no soap or caustics. It carries a natural inbuilt anesthetic and astringent found in white oak bark itself. The natural healing power of oak bark as an herb is renowned. The cleanser flushes out deeply embedded impurities and acts as a disencrustant, which means it removes the hardened sebum oils, dry skin, dead epithelial cells and toxins.

Both the White Oak Cleanser and the White Oak Liquid Cleansing Creme are water soluble, containing stearic acid and oleic acid, which are found naturally in human skin. Their polarized water contains many vitamins and minerals from herbs. They both contain PCMX, which is an anti fungus, a full spectrum antiseptic, germicide and mold inhibitor. They contain no soap, dyes, chemicals or perfumes. Totally pure from the bark of oak trees. More about them in the last chapter.

You should occasionally use a rough textured washcloth with the liquid Cleanser, or just splash off with warm (never hot) water, followed by many cold splashes. Never use facial tissues, for they contain infinitesimal wood splinters which irritate and damage the skin. Always apply a moisturizer immediately. Consider *Fanie's Fine Line Creme* or *Apricot Creme* followed by her special *Mineral Spray*, which acts as a toner, refreshing astringent and additional moisturizer — or consider a product called *Vita Balm*, which is an excellent under make-up moisturizer sold by Patricia Allison. When I'm staying home all day without make-up I use the Fine Line or Apricot Creme. If I'm in a hurry to apply my make-up I use Vita Balm. Either way, use Fanie's Mineral Spray or a spray of good mineral water.

Whether you use bar soap, liquid cleanser, or cleansing cream, you may wish to steam your face before or after cleansing. Apply a hot washcloth and hold it against your face a few minutes. Steaming opens the pores and draws all the dirt and oils to the surface. After steaming and cleansing, splash your face either with warm water or use an abrasive cotton washcloth, the better to remove the top layer of cells and the updrawn impurities. Follow with a cold water splash, then add a moisturizer. You can't begin too early to add a moisturizer to your skin. All skins need moisturizers, especially dry and normal skin. Although oily skin requires very little, mature skin requires even more moisturizing. All skins need it after washing the face. Do massage well (with upward strokes) so that it is fully absorbed rather than drying on the surface. Pay attention to the throat and around the eyes, and follow with a mineral water spray.

Occasionally a moisturizer will cause a rash. Many contain parabens, which are used to fight fungus and bacteria. Some people are allergic to the parabens. If your skin develops a rash after using your moisturizer, check the label. If it contains parabens, test for a possible allergy. I'll tell you later how to test.

Men, use a moisturizer after shaving. Ladies, every opportunity. Avoid any product containing glycerin or any other humectant. Glycerin absorbs moisture even from your skin. Thus, instead of moisturizing as it is supposed to do, if the air is dry the glycerin, seeking moisture, will absorb it from the cells of your skin. Avoid! Avoid moisturizers containing mineral oil, which only lubricates and seals the skin surface. Choose brands containing amino acids and vitamins —

preferably with vegetable or fruit oils, such as avocado, apricot, sesame, wheat germ, etc. If you unexpectedly run out of your favorite moisturizer, never fear — almond oil to the rescue, right out of your kitchen. Or sesame oil, or olive oil. Of course, they're cold pressed from the health store, aren't they? If all else fails, apply a slice of avocado, right from the refrigerator. Or rub a slice of cucumber over your face. Also avoid bath powder altogether. It "clogs" the skin, preventing natural "breathing" of the pores. Not only that, it's filled with undesirable ingredients.

Choose refreshing lotions and astringents carefully, since many contain dangerous chemicals, dyes and fragrances which, if used regularly, rob the skin of natural moisture, enlarge pores and create altogether undesirable results. Natural plant-derivative liquid cleansers contain natural astringents. An excellent refreshing lotion which contains plant derivatives is Patricia Allison's *Wild Fern Freshener*. It's a mild refreshing lotion containing alfalfa extract, vitamin E and essential oil — absolutely no harsh chemicals. Or you may want to mix your own, using 1 oz. of cider vinegar to 3 oz. of distilled water. Or add lemon juice to your rinse water. Either restores the acid mantle to your skin. Or you may prefer Fanie's Mineral Spray which acts as an astringent and also as a moisturizer.

Sleep with a contoured pillow. A fat pillow raises the head unnaturally, often wrinkling the throat and causing puffy skin. Chiropractors and osteopaths usually offer a special contoured pillow for their clients, specially structured to provide support for the neck to relieve cervical or neck pain and tension, which often leads to headaches, throat problems, and sometimes

shoulder pain and tingling in the fingers, as well as
wrinkles on the face. You may wish to order a special
pillow from my personal chiropractor, Dr. Noll Walker.
The pillow has a hollow center for the head yet
maintains support for the neck. Since sleeping on this
contoured pillow I've seldom experienced a headache,
which were frequent previously. He is also distributor
of remarkable oriental products called *Sunrider*. They
offer an excellent face cream which is extremely
effective for tightening the skin and eliminating
wrinkles. It *really* does! For full information for the
pillow and the Sunrider products, contact Dr. Walker
personally. (Address elsewhere).

Some prefer a tiny baby pillow filled with soft
goosedown. One choice is presently available from
Hammacher Schlemmer, who call it their travel pillow.
Or from Solutions. (Addresses elsewhere). Hammacher
Schlemmer also presently carries what they call the
Wrinkle-Reducing pillow, which reduces wrinkles by
eliminating pressure on your face and neck. It also has
a hollow center for the head. Write for information.
They also offer an ultrasonic humidifier that is quiet
enough for your bedroom — a whirlpool bathtub spa for
home use (I have one, it's marvelous) — a tiny facial
sauna that emits a mighty stream of steam, also good
for traveling. J.C. Penney's catalog also offers a Kaz
facial sauna that is great.

The skin is, in itself, a vibrant, living, growing
organ — your largest organ. The epidermal deep
"mother" cells regenerate and form "daughter" cells
which push the elder cells outward to the surface of the
skin, where they "die," creating a rough surface. This
is a continuing process. The surface cells are usually

denied a needed supply of water and other nutrients, which results in the death of the cells. The face of a man often appears younger than that of a woman the same age. The daily shave is believed to be the cause — the daily removal of dead surface cells plus the automatic facial exercises performed. Since women do not shave it is necessary to find other methods of dead cell removal. It is possible to aid nature in this sloughing off process, and the freshness and youth of facial skin depends upon it.

Steaming the face helps. A facial sauna is great, or simply apply a steaming hot washcloth. Or boil a pot or teakettle of water on the stove. Then remove it to a table at the proper height for bending your face over the steam. Place a towel over your head, forming a tent to cover both your face and the steam. Hold your face about ten inches from the kettle, allowing the steam to rise into the face, softening and rehydrating the skin. I take advantage of our humidifier, which I keep operating constantly to make sure we have moisture in the house. I pause frequently and hold my face directly in the stream of moist spray.

Those with dry and lined complexions may wish to follow the steaming with a hot oil treatment and massage. Warm about a tablespoon of wheat germ oil in a small container (not aluminum). Allow it to warm, not to boil, as overheating would destroy the natural vitamins E and A in the wheat germ. Now massage the oil into your dry skin, tensing the muscles and using upward strokes. The vitamin E in the wheat germ oil will aid in erasing age lines, especially the fine lines around the eyes.

Investigate the use of enzymes as a potent catalyst

for sloughing off surface cells. Most should be left on at least five minutes to allow the enzyme action to "digest" the dead cells. Or you may prefer scrubbing with moistened cornmeal or oatmeal. There are other products now available in addition to those already mentioned. A special textured facial washcloth helps, or use a 100% cotton washcloth. Special creams, such as the almond scrub, are available if you prefer. Patricia Allison offers an excellent almond and honey *Swedish Scrub* that is so gentle it can be used daily. Or you may prefer *Fanie's Unveil Skin Peel*, which contains hydroxypropyl methylcellulose and phenol. It's perfect for removing the cells, resulting in a slight skin peel. It can be used daily or at least twice a week, to help keep your skin supplied with fresh "daughter" cells. More about these products in a later chapter.

Oily skin should be blotted occasionally with astringent lotion. Wear your hair off your face. Oil from your hair, mixed with facial oil, could cause blemishes. Dab your face occasionally with apple juice. Or with sour milk. Leave on several minutes, then rinse off.

If possible, sleep with a humidifier in the bedroom to keep the skin moist. For humidifying throughout the house, put a pan of water on your stove or radiator. And consider keeping water in your bathtub. The circulating currents of hot or cool air from your heater or air conditioner will be saturated with moisture throughout the house. Or place water near the hot air vents in each room as air blowing over the surface will absorb and vaporize the water, which will counteract skin dryness. And drink plenty of water. More about humidifiers in Chapter Three.

Facial Masks

Usually one chooses between two basic masks — the gel mask or the pack mask. The pack masks are those that dry and crust over the skin, drawing it tight. Those with dry or more aged complexions should choose the gel mask. Those with normal or oily complexions should choose the pack mask. The familiar clay mask is a good example of a crusting pack mask, since it absorbs oil from the skin. Women with dry or lined skin should avoid the clay or mud mask or use it sparingly. It may be used occasionally for deep cleansing and exfoliation of dead skin cells. Patricia Allison has a truly unique herbal mask — *Babyskin Masque* — that can be used on all skin types. The active ingredients are vegetable gum and aromatic balsam. It refines pores, stimulates circulation, and sloughs off dead dry cells. She also offers a peppermint gel mask which can be used daily, that moisturizes and stimulates.

Or you may prefer *Fanie's Facial Mask*. It's a dry powder which must be mixed with a special liquid or water to form a combination of the gel-pack mask. It dries to a crust, but is excellent for both dry or oily skin. It's incredible. Applied in a test to only half the face, results can be seen immediately. It's not essential but you may first apply Fanie's Unveil Skin Peel. Let it dry a few moments if you can spare the time. Now mix the mask powder with *Fanie's Tru-Skin Lotion* or water and apply the mask over the Skin Peel. If possible lie down and relax, preferably on a slant board, soak in a warm tub bath, watch TV, or read a book. As the mask firms, it is rehydrating the skin from deep within its own cells. The mask is preventing evaporation. It is also absorbing deeply lodged dirt and debris. The tightening of the mask provides the skin with a temporary lift.

According to the late Clyde Johnson, their chemist, Fanie's Mask is the only one available which can be applied directly over the eyes. He said its contents are so pure it can do no damage to the delicate eye tissues. It aids in preventing wrinkles around the eyes. Try to soak in a tub bath at least once a week — and apply your mask at that time. After removing the mask, follow with Fanie's Mineral Spray or a spray of your choice. Last, apply a good moisturizer to face and throat, perhaps Patricia Allison's Vita Balm. Later at bedtime, apply Beleza's honey/vitamin/mineral Anti-Aging Cream, one of Fanie's night creams, or a cream of your choice. There are many available — especially the Retin-A creams and alpha hydroxy fruit acids. More about these later.

If the facial mask you use requires avoiding the eye area, why not simultaneously apply a treatment to the eyes. Make a tea of rosemary, camomile, fennel, or eyebright. Add one tablespoon of herbs to four ounces of boiling water. Steep a few minutes in a covered container, strain and cool in refrigerator. Or purchase tea bags for making tea — camomile tea bags would be an excellent choice. After applying the facial mask, dip cotton pats in the cold tea and apply to the closed eyes while lying on a slant board or reclining on the bed with the feet ten to fifteen inches higher than the head. Be sure to purchase pure cotton pats or balls of cotton wool. Avoid the use of synthetic cotton balls or pats.

Wrinkles! Wrinkles!

The Cause of Wrinkles — There is far more to skin wrinkles than aging. The very youthful begin laying the foundation for wrinkles by daily bad habits. Just to name a few: failure to cleanse the skin regularly (never retire without cleansing the skin and applying a moisturizer, regardless of your age), overdoses of sun which shrivel and age it; and poor circulation, since the blood must carry the proper nutrients to the cells. A major cause is a faulty diet — fast foods, soft drinks, fatty foods (animal fats), fried foods, processed foods, all contribute; overheated homes and offices; bad facial expressions; arid and high winds; failure to use the best moisturizer; failure to drink plenty of water to hydrate the skin.

The pH Factor — Do be aware of the "acid mantle" or the normal state of acidity of the skin. The scale of measuring the degree of acidity is called the pH scale and the gauge runs from zero to fourteen. From one to seven represents total acidity. Total alkalinity registers from seven to fourteen. The ideal range for the skin on the pH scale is from 4.5 to 5.5. This slightly acid state is required to shield the skin from bacteria, fungi and other contaminations. The pH claim on many labels implies a pH balance, but it simply doesn't mean that it's acid balanced. Even though most cosmetic manufacturers are aware of the importance of the pH factor, cosmetics are seldom created with this in mind. A cream or moisturizer ranging from 4.5 to 5.5 pH is ideal. Do try to select such a moisturizer. Test it by using a strip of litmus or nitrazine paper, available at your drug or health store.

The urine should also register acid on the pH scale. It can also be tested through the use of litmus or nitrazine paper. A small strip of the paper, exposed to urine, will turn yellow to indicate acidity, or purple to indicate alkalinity. The package of litmus paper will provide the pH scale of measurement. The ideal acid state of urine is 5.5. If it registers far into the purple alkaline state, it can be restored to its normal acidity by mixing two teaspoons of honey and two teaspoons of apple cider vinegar in a cup of water. Drink this "cocktail" for several days, or daily, to maintain the normal acid state. When the urine is not slightly acid, the body itself is less able to resist bacterial invasions — both from within and without.

Retin-A and Retinol-A — are hailed as wrinkle removers. And they certainly are! The difference is: *Retin-A* contains tretinoin, a substance which has been known to damage some skins. Therefore it must be prescribed by a doctor. *Retinol-A*, a different formula, can be purchased over the counter or ordered by mail. Clyde Johnson, in the Fanie Laboratory, produced a rare and marvelous Retinol-A — by incorporating modified vitamin A into a special transderma formula allowing for a chemically balanced product. This means that the resorcin and vitamin A in the formula have been combined with moisturizers to combat any damage while effectively removing wrinkles. The bottle clearly warns that a patch test should be observed. Clyde Johnson's Retinol-A formula (Fanie's) may be the only one presently available which has moisturizers carefully balancing the vitamin A. Should you purchase elsewhere, make very sure the formula contains moisturizers — natural, if possible. Karie Hayden,

R.C., Fanie's distributor listed in the last chapter, declares Fanie's Retinol-A Creme to be well tolerated, safe and effective.

Another source for Retinol-A is E. Burnham Co. (address elsewhere). I'm not sure what is in Burnham's formula so cannot enlighten you. But don't order from firms that don't offer a money-back guarantee. I ordered a jar from a certain well-known company whose cream certainly did *not* remove anything — so I returned it and asked for a refund. They refused to return my money, saying their products were so excellent no return was ever given. But Fanie's products *all* carry a money-back guarantee, as do Burnham's. But be aware of the difference between Retinol-A and Retin-A cream. The Retinol-A released by Fanie does not contain tretinoin, the chemical in Retin-A. Retin-A, with tretinoin, has been known to cause redness, blistering, severe local swelling, and sensitivity to sunlight. Nevertheless, unless you have an allergic reaction, it's great. It certainly does remove wrinkles and results should be within a month. Have your doctor prescribe it for you so that he can monitor the results.

Years ago I heard of Retin-A — long before the present popular craze. It was very successful for me, but only because I worked out my own personal "treatment." I applied the Retin-A after my bath early in the evening. Then at bedtime several hours later, I applied Beleza Anti-Aging Cream. By the time I completed my prayers (which I always say at bedtime), I could stroke away all the scaly surface skin, using upward strokes of course. I would repeat the upward massaging the following morning, following Sanford Bennett's method. If I used the Retin-A without removing the dead cells with Beleza, it didn't work. All it did was dry out and wrinkle my skin. If you're having problems with Retinol or Retin-A, you may wish to try this or a similar treatment.

Oriental Pearl Cream — Shortly before press time I discovered an extraordinary new moisturizing face cream that reduces lines and wrinkles, making your skin look radiant and more youthful. It is a most unique blend of rare Chinese herbs and crushed pearls ground into a fine powder. Even though I've only been using it for a relatively short time, the remarkable results are quite apparent. For more information or to order, see Chapter 10 for address.

Other Wrinkle Removers — Try egg white, beaten, applied to the face and allowed to harden. Then rinse off with warm water. Don't leave it on too long. Egg whites left on over ten minutes can be harmful. Or try Patricia Allison's *Un-Line*, a nonsurgical "facelift." Its active ingredient is extracted from a rare sea plant. It also contains mountain ash berry extract.

Acupuncture and Acupressure Facelifts — Again, see *The Book of Beginning Again*. Observe the face chart near the back of the book. Try applying pressure on the points designated once a day for about a month, then a couple of times a week. Hold the pressure on each point for about one minute. The results are amazing! Also be aware of facelifts via acupuncture. Master Sehan Kim of Los Angeles, mentioned in *Beginning Again*, still gives them. He can be contacted at the address given in the last chapter.

Chemical Face Peels — given by plastic or cosmetic surgeons, are extremely effective but be cautious. They are *not* painless because the chemical applied is a controlled acid burn, the purpose being to destroy the top layer of skin. Applied usually with a cotton applicator, each "touch" burns for several seconds, then it settles into a stinging sensation much like a mild sunburn. Then your face and throat are usually covered with a material which keeps moisture over the skin for several days. The procedure can be done in a doctor's office, but afterward one must remain secluded for about ten days for the healing process. The new skin is pink and lovely, many wrinkles gone. But the skin remains extremely sensitive to sun rays afterward, for at least six months. Exposure is to be totally avoided. Also the risks involved are skin infections, cold sores, and keloids. A keloid is a strange hard bump under the skin that needs to be surgically removed.

I've just heard of a new type of peel that is not the usual chemical formula — of interest to folks living in Southern California. Dr. Robert Harmon, who performs the procedure in his office in Palm Desert (near Palm Springs) states that the formula contains no harsh chemicals. He says he has never known it to produce keloids or sun sensitivity. The after-effects are truly amazing. If interested, see Chapter 10 for Dr. Harmon's address and phone number.

Laser Resurfacing — Comes word of a new high-tech skin treatment that is reputed to remove the outer leathery skin of the face and throat to restore beauty. It is said to vanquish wrinkles altogether, banishing the appearance of old age. Almost too good to be true. The process involves laser beams. It has been developed by Dr. Lawrence M. David, a former instructor at USC in Los Angeles, and presently director of the Hermosa Skin Medical Clinic, address elsewhere. Dr. David states the procedure is without pain because lasers seal the nerve endings, and patients can return to normal activities within a few hours. Dr. David emphasizes the treatment requires a specially trained surgeon. Write him direct for information regarding such a surgeon in your area. (See the last chapter.)

Novadermy Live Cell Therapy — I'm happy to tell you of a skin rejuvenation technique called Novadermy, which uses live cell transplants. Once available only in exclusive clinics in Europe, it has now been brought to this continent and is available just over the border from San Diego, California, in Tijuana, Mexico. The beautiful clinic there, called *Genesis West*, also offers live cell injections, which are renowned for regenerating the body. You'll be told more about that in a later chapter.

Novadermy, for the face, claims incredible results. It's neither facelifting nor peeling in the usual sense. It's a proven medical procedure employing whole, live, fetal cells that, without pain or surgery, permanently replace aged skin with a virgin mantle of vital young cells. Whereas the usual skin peel uses chemical applications of a phenolic acid solution which sometimes proves unsatisfactory, Novadermy uses a combination of herbal and carbolate solutions. After the outer skin is removed, it is then covered by a suspension of live fetal cells which gradually integrate into a new cellular structure free of wrinkles and blemishes. If interested, seek more information through Genesis West's American representative at VitaChem International, Inc., address elsewhere. Of course, if you are opposed to any involvement of animal use in cosmetics, you'll not want to consider this.

Chapter Three

God-Made Beautifiers and Guidelines

"Kitchen" and natural remedies for keeping the face young should be of equal interest to both men and women. They require very little time and manifest amazing results.

A Yogurt and Sour Milk Skin Peel — Apply yogurt, apple juice or sour milk to your face and throat to remove the glue-like surface of the skin. Wrinkles vanish, dry scaly patches of skin disappear, age spots fade, and acne is healed. So say the latest releases from skin specialists. Good heavens! — my Mama used buttermilk constantly on her skin to keep it "fair!" Wonder where she got the idea!

Yogurt can also be added to your douche water, ladies, to keep the vagina acid. Add just enough water to yogurt to make the yogurt fluid. Apply yogurt directly on an itchy vulva or rectal area and cover with a light sanitary napkin. Repeat every two hours.

An Apple Facelift — New medical findings prove the effectiveness of apple acids on the skin. Apples contain natural chemicals called *alpha hydroxy acids* — or AHA — that removes wrinkles and the dead cells on the surface skin. Dermatologists are now developing a prescription cream containing AHA, but you can make your own at home:

Make a thick apple sauce with peeled apples and milk. Cook until soft, then thoroughly blend the formula. Apply to your face and throat. Leave it on for from 15 to 30 minutes unless the acids are too strong for your skin. Apply once a week or as often as your skin will tolerate it. The AHA plus the malic acid in the apple accomplishes a slow natural chemical peel. But do test the treatment for allergic reaction before applying to your face — a patch test on the inner arm, near the elbow. Such a slow peel may require the better part of a year. Just as this manuscript was going to press, I discovered a new product called *New Feeling* which can be purchased at health stores. It's based on AHA and is supposed to be marvelous! It has only recently become available. Try it! Other suggestions follow:

1. Slice a cucumber into your blender. Mix it at high speed until it liquifies. Strain it and apply the liquid.

2. Tartaric acid, found in wine, also acts as a face peel. To correct oily skin problems try white wine applied with a pure cotton pat, for light-skinned people. Red wine for brunettes and olive-skinned. It should be repeated about once every two weeks.

3. Half and half lemon juice and water is excellent, but try it first for its potency. If lemon is too strong, add more water. The lemon contains salicylic acid as well as citric acid. It will also peel the face. The acids in oranges, grape-

fruit, pineapple, papaya, lemons, apples, grapes and cucumbers are excellent to create a wrinkle-free skin, causing the top layer of dead cells to slough off and leave the face fresh and youthful. The malic acid in apples is what accomplishes the peel. Tartaric acid in grapes and citric acid in citrus and other fruits are the cause of the peeling. Mix any of these juices with water, sour milk, buttermilk or sour cream before applying. Sour milk is excellent because of its lactic acid. Use cautiously until you discover how sensitive your skin might be to these powerful natural beautifiers. Add any of the juices of these fruits or milk to your bath water to freshen and purify the skin of your body — one fourth of a cup to an entire tub. To simply rinse your face, add a tablespoon of these fruit juices to a basin of lukewarm water. Be sure your eyes are closed. And follow immediately with a clear water rinse.

The Mayonnaise Treatment — Some people swear by mayonnaise as a skin treatment. First steam the face by applying a hot washcloth. Then massage the mayonnaise gently but thoroughly into the skin and allow it to penetrate, since it possesses all kinds of protein and skin food. It should remain from 10 to 15 minutes. Then remove with warm water followed by a moisturizer, then Fanie's Mineral Spray or mineral water of your choice.

A Fine Facial Astringent — To repeat, many astringents are damaging for facial use. They certainly should be used only on oily skin. Refreshing lotion should be used on all other skin types. Try applying a slice of fresh tomato as an astringent for oily skin. Fanie's Mineral Spray may be used as a mild astringent for all types of skin. Spray after cleansing, before make-up, after make-up, and all through the day, right on top of make-up. It keeps the make-up fresh and simultaneously feeds the skin nourishment.

Remember, too, Patricia Allison's Wild Fern Freshener with its alfalfa extract and lemon oil.

Honey and Beauty — Honey has been used as a natural moisturizer for centuries. But it is far more than that. It will also lift off dead skin cells. Be sure it's thin and be sure it's raw. Add lemon juice if you wish, but don't leave it on more than fifteen minutes. It will restore the natural acid mantle of your skin. Elsewhere, you'll read of the effect of lemon in erasing wrinkles. Or beat an egg yolk and add it to honey. Remove after five or ten minutes. It's the honey in Beleza's Anti-Aging Formula which helps make it such an excellent night cream — plus all the vitamins and minerals.

Mask — Kaolin, available at health stores in powdered form, makes a good home mask. With added water or Fanie's Tru-Skin, it becomes a clay mask. If your skin is oily, add a few drops of lemon juice.

Vitamin E as a Beauty Treatment — Vitamin E has long been known as an excellent natural moisturizer for the skin and has been so used in creams and lotions. But now it is beginning to be recognized as equally beneficial to increase skin elasticity. Also, vitamin E oil rubbed over cuts and minor burns appears to be extremely beneficial. It also has an anti-inflammatory and wound healing effect on the skin, especially for diminishing scars. It protects delicate membranes of cells whether taken internally or applied topically. Acne medications almost always contain vitamin E because it decreases redness and soreness. It's also now being applied with finger massage to bleeding gums and gum infections. It's being incorporated into sun burn preventive medications because evidence shows it to be effective for blocking ultraviolet rays and helping prevent skin cancer. Corn, cottonseed, and soybean oil contain

high portions of vitamin E. Also wheat germ oil and butter. Taken as a vitamin, seek a natural source from your
health store because it remains active in the body much
longer than the synthetic forms. The usual daily intake
is 400 IUs.

Youth and Health Baths — Avoid long baths, both winter and summer. Twenty minutes is sufficient. Soaking
in plain water dries your skin. Add bath oil or herbs to
counteract drying, available at health stores. Or add
Fanie's Sweet Birch Body Cleanser to your bath. Use it
instead of soap in your shower. It is chemical free and has
the most amazing healing properties. It's made from nettle, kelp, sweet birch and hydroprophomethyl-cellulose.
This deep pore natural bark cleanser does not leave a
residue on the skin. Its astringent is naturally contained
in sweet birch. Adding a capful to your tub soak changes
it to a healing experience. It heals sores and irritations
as well as cleanses, just by soaking in it. Occasionally add
a squirt of Fanie's Oak Bark Cleanser to obtain the healing
effects of natural oak bark. Excellent, too, are mineral
salts from the Dead Sea, available at health stores. Or try
a capful of Patricia Allison's Vita Balm with a capful of
her Roman Oil Beauty Bath. It works in the hardest of
waters and its oils truly alleviate dry itching skin. Fanie's
and Allison's both are more God-made than man-made.
Avoid drug store bubble baths. Too many dangerous chemicals. Again, never use bath powder after baths. Use body
oils and moisturizers instead.

To counteract radiation effects of x-rays, soak for twenty minutes in a full tub of water to which you've added two
cups of baking soda and two cups of Epsom salts, or non-
iodized salt from your health store. One should soak as
soon as possible following an x-ray. Repeat it twice a week

for a month. If you can tolerate it, stir one teaspoon of sea salt and one teaspoon of baking soda in one quart of water and drink one glass while soaking in the tub. Add the rest to your tub water. A soda-salt tub soak could be taken once a week continuously to neutralize radiation fall-out absorbed through the skin and breath. It is also very healing. Avoid too hot water, try tepid instead. Shower no more than once a day and follow all baths with a moisturizing body lotion. Patricia Allison's *Petalskin Balm* is excellent. Her natural formulas are great for smooth, blemish-free body skin.

Add milk to your tub soak. Use powdered milk if you choose, as it may be less expensive. Be sure to rinse in a shower afterward. Otherwise the remaining milk film could irritate the skin.

To aid circulation, add a cup of white wine to your tub soak. To make all your tub soaks more effective, add four ounces of sesame oil. Your skin will feel great.

The Benefits of Lemon

God must have made the lemon specially for the well-being of mankind, and for beauty as well. The list of benefits is extensive and I must emphasize them:

A. After cleansing the skin, apply lemon juice with a cotton pat or stroke the face and neck gently with lemon peel, making sure not to scratch the skin with the peel. This restores the natural pH acid mantle and acts as a natural moisturizer. If your skin is too sensitive to allow the lemon juice to dry, apply and rinse immediately until the skin becomes accustomed to the treatment. Otherwise allow it to dry, which will require probably ten or fifteen minutes.

The lemon juice will bleach out freckles, blemishes, heal acne pimples and blackheads, reduce pores, and remove the surface skin with its wrinkles. Rinse off with warm water and splash with cold, then apply a moisturizer. Apply only once a week in the beginning. After a few weeks, apply twice a week, then work up to a daily treatment. If full strength is intolerable, dilute with milk, sour milk or water. Or apply a formula of three ounces of lemon juice to five drops of pure glycerin, the only time glycerin is advisable. Or add olive oil to the lemon juice.

B. Fingers stained with cigarettes or vegetable coloring may be bleached by rubbing with lemon peel.

C. To strengthen the fingernails and soften the cuticle, apply lemon juice daily.

D. Lemon juice mixed with olive or almond oil is especially effective in removing blackheads. Steam the face thoroughly with a hot washcloth. Once you have drawn blood to the face, massage it gently with the lemon juice-oil mixture, then, using a washcloth and White Oak Cleanser, scrub the face thoroughly but gently. Follow with another warm steaming and finish with a cold water splash. Apply a moisturizer.

E. Apply to brown spots and freckles. It often will fade them after a few weeks. Apply with pure cotton balls or cotton-tipped applicators. If you have sensitive or problem skin, always consult a doctor or dermatologist before using any of these suggestions.

Guidelines

Dermatitis — Dermatitis is an inflamed itching, scaling and crusting of the skin. Try castor oil, Fanie's Herbal Oil, aloe vera gel, or *Allison's Ultra-Rich* containing jojoba oil and vitamin E.

Castor Oil — Try this natural remedy for almost everything. Drop five drops of cold pressed castor oil under the tongue daily. It's been known to heal allergies and it certainly slowly detoxifies the system. For all purposes, use only cold pressed castor oil, obtainable from Drs. Gladys and William McGarey's A.R.E. Clinic in Phoenix, Cayce Corner (address elsewhere). Time and time again the Drs. McGarey have healed serious afflictions using a castor oil pack, which was highly recommended by the famous psychic healer Edgar Cayce. You'll find much more about this incredible product in *The You Book: A Treasury of Health and Healing.**

Insect Bites and Bee Stings — Try ice cubes. Also apply unseasoned meat tenderizer mixed with water. My mother always dabbed our ant bites with bluing, the kind she used to bleach clothes. Try applying the papaya fruit.

Humidifiers — During the winter months the skin of your face and body may become dried and chapped. The skin is ravaged by artificial heat in homes and offices which makes the air extremely dry. The air currents keep moving past your skin, which further dries it. Both dry and oily skin become dry and flaky when the humidity is low. You need excess moisture in the air. Purchase a humidifier, or place a small container of water in each room.

Use a humidifier in the bedroom. Avoid using tap water in the humidifier — it's loaded with all sorts of chemicals and metals, such as asbestos, lead, aluminum, and many environmental pollutants which should not be inhaled. Use distilled water. Or purchase steam or cool-

*Order from Astara, 800 W. Arrow Hwy., P.O. Box 5003, Upland, CA 91785

mist humidifiers. It's extremely important that the water be changed in all humidifiers daily to avoid a buildup of bacteria which, inhaled, could result in recurring sore throats. They should be cleaned with vinegar water each week without fail.

Combating the Elements — Keep the temperature in your home as low as you comfortably can. Avoid standing or sitting near open fireplaces. It may sound romantic to sit dreaming by a lovely warm fireplace, but this is the type of heat that most quickly extracts moisture from the skin leaving it dry and even itchy.

Switch to cotton underclothes. The skin can breathe through the natural fibers. Synthetic fabrics cause itching and chapping, and the pores cannot discharge toxins. Drink more liquids — water, herb teas, juices.

Use a liquid or cream cleansing lotion, never soap, during the winter months. Switch to an oilier moisturizer, and never leave home without it. Do be aware that you need a sunscreen even in winter. Snow magnifies the sun's glare and destructive ultraviolet rays. Do change to deeper colors in your make-up. The skin tends to pale and the shades you use during summer may need to be intensified. Keep lipstick or a lip balm on your lips to prevent chapping. Spray your face often with Mineral Spray or distilled water — even over your make-up.

If you are a runner, do not run in cold weather for many reasons; but for purposes of protecting the skin, change to walking. Skin loses moisture when the air currents are in motion. Even while walking, cover your hands and legs. They're vulnerable to cold. Before coming indoors from the cold, pause and warm your cheeks and nose with your hands. This will avoid the risk of abrupt temperature changes causing broken capillaries, often called spider veins.

Your Skin and the Sun

Avoid the sun. Energy from the sun has a spectrum of many different wavelengths. The longer infrared rays register as heat and the shorter rays register as light. In the light rays are found the short ultraviolet rays, radiating intense energy. It is the longer ultraviolet heat rays that burn — the burn equaling that of a radiation burn — and it's these rays that are most potent and injurious between the hours of 10:00 a.m. to 3:00 p.m. Patricia Allison's literature says it even better:

"Dermatologists have long known that the sun's ultraviolet (UV) rays damage the skin. We feel it is important that everyone knows the facts about the sun's effect on the skin, and once knowing, act! Recent findings indicate that there are two types of UV rays involved in the destructive process (UVA and UVB).

"UVA rays penetrate deep into the skin. These rays eventually alter the tissues (the dermis) that give the skin its structure, thus causing wrinkles. Almost all wrinkles are caused by this process. The UVA rays attack the skin year-round from dawn to dusk.

"UVB rays are more powerful than the UVA rays. They cause sunburn and peeling of the outer layer of the skin (the epidermis), and are believed to be the cause of skin cancer. These rays are more abundant in the summer months, between 10:00 a.m. and 3:00 p.m., and get stronger the further south you live. The earth's protective ozone layer filters out many of these rays, but with the damage being done to the ozone layer itself, scientists are predicting that we will see a much higher percentage of skin cancer in the future. Fair, easily sunburned persons, are more at risk than dark skinned persons."

Actually, exposure to the sun's ultraviolet rays is exposure to radiation. Those taking tranquilizers, antibacterial agents in medical soaps, drugs to control high blood pressure, antibiotics, diuretics, estrogen or diabetic medication should particularly avoid sunshine. Also perfumes or colognes should never be worn during exposure to the sun. Suntanning quickly dries out the skin, creating a leathery look. It destroys the collagen and elastin components of the skin, and causes the melanin to come up — which is the substance in the skin causing the skin to tan. The sun's damage is rapid and accumulative although the damage done may not appear for several years. That skin cancer is one result is well known. A sure sign of skin cancer is an eruption or a sore that does not heal. It continues to bleed, then scab and bleed again. Also beware of a freckle that suddenly grows larger, or a wart or red scaly patch of skin or mole that manifests a sudden change.

Avoid suntanning parlors like the plague! They claim their sunning lamps shield out most of the harmful ultraviolet rays and leave only the rays that do not damage, but don't you believe it! It simply isn't true. As a healer, I've seen many tears shed by women begging for prayers to heal the many facial skin cancers caused by sun lamps! Dreadful! And they believed the lamps were safe. One precious friend had forty skin cancers removed from her face, and more were forming. Her face was scarred, she had also developed cataracts. All because of sun lamps.

Once the skin is damaged, the harm can rarely be undone. So do wear a sunhat, or carry an umbrella, and apply a sunscreen cream at least an hour before exposure if possible. Some dermatologists advise against a sunscreen with PABA. They say it clogs pores, attracts dust and other irritants from the atmosphere and thus contributes to skin cancer. But it's controversial. You may prefer to use products containing PABA. Consider Patricia Allison's *Nutrient Balm Sun Screen* (SPF 15) that protects from both wrinkle causing and cancer causing rays — with no PABA. Or use Fanie's Sateen Velvet Lotion which contains a 17 sunscreen. There is another new sunscreen on the market now that blocks both the UVA rays and the UVB rays. It's called *Photoplex*, made by Herbert Laboratories. And do use aloe vera gel in case of a sunburn. Cloudy days are equally as dangerous as sunny because the radiation of sun rays can penetrate and burn without sunlight. Sitting under an umbrella helps, but radiation rays strike from all angles and beach sand reflects them — so at all times, when exposed to the summer sun, protect your skin.

If you insist on tanning, begin at least a week before your tanning program to take the following supplements: vitamin C (3000 mg. a day), vitamin E (400 units a day), Selenium (250 mg. daily), PABA (500 mg twice a day), Beta-carotene (15-30 mg. daily). If you have a history of kidney or liver problems, hepatitis or diabetes, consult your doctor before taking these supplements. If you are a smoker be equally cautious. Begin with ten minutes of tanning a day and work up to longer. At all times wear a sunscreen. Remember, water reflects rays, especially near a beach, so be cautious. To repeat, the hours to avoid are between 10:00 a.m. and 3:00 p.m., when the incoming ultraviolet rays are at the height of their burning power.

Never lie motionless in the burning sunshine during these five hours. The rays of the sun will pierce any protection, whether a sunblocking agent or any other cream.

Those who insist upon a suntan really accelerate the rate of aging. By age forty, the foolish suntanner will look sixty. Once there was very little one could do to correct the damage once it was done, but there are now available skin treatments which might help, such as live cell therapy, mentioned in Chapter Two. Or laser treatments, also mentioned earlier. It's possible Retin-A may offer some help toward erasing the premature wrinkles. See a dermatologist. In their skin therapy centers across the nation, Fanie offers deep tissue and deep cell treatments which benefit all skin problems, including the folds of wrinkles caused by sun damage. (See last chapter). Needless to say, the suntanned person is risking an almost certain problem of skin cancer. Although skin cancer is seldom life threatening, it certainly can be devastating to a youthful appearance.

Suntanning and AIDS — And now, to add a resounding warning, a late news release reports that exposure to sunlight actually triggers the AIDS virus! If a virus is lying in a dormant state, direct exposure to the sun could activate the virus into life- threatening status. The same is true of the suntanning lamps. It's the harmful ultraviolet rays that cause the transformation. This timely report comes from Dr. Louis Qualtiere, a microbiologist at the University of Saskatchewan in Canada.

Citrus and Sunbathing — Avoid eating citrus fruits while in the sun. The oil in the peel of an orange, lemon, or lime creates a sensitivity to your lips, causing them to be more sensitive to the sun. You can thus end up with badly sunburned lips. When exposed to the sun, it's safer to sip good mineral water.

Sunbathing and the Wrist Meter— Consider wearing a wrist meter which can eliminate the dangers of sunburn. It's a device marketed by researchers at the Temple University Skin and Cancer Hospital in Philadelphia. Called a *dosimeter*, it's worn like a wrist watch. It measures sun-burning and cancer-causing ultraviolet radiation. When the skin has absorbed a safe amount of the sun's radiations, an alarm goes off warning that the skin is receiving too many dangerous rays. The device is battery powered. Soon on the market, too, is a special bandage which, taped on the skin, turns blue to warn the wearer it's time to leave the sun.

For Sunparched Dry Skin— Apply aloe vera gel, Fanie's Protein Creme, or Allison's Vita Balm.

Sunburn— Wrap crushed ice in a washcloth and rub gently over burned area, or just place it securely. Apply aloe vera gel, preferably directly from the leaf of the plant. Or blend fresh cucumber into milk in your blender and allow it to soak for five to six hours, then apply the mixture to the burn. Or add a pinch of baking soda to half a cup of milk and pat it into the sunburned area. Or use Fanie's Protein Creme. It contains vitamin E and isolated soya protein which helps skin to heal quickly. Take a cool bath with four tablespoons of baking soda and a cup of milk added to the bath water. This temporarily alkalizes your skin. Or soak in a tepid tub to which a pint of any herb tea is added. Dry the skin and apply aloe vera or Calamine Ointment.

Many common and widely advertised cosmetic products do more harm than good and may actually be dangerous — products such as sunburn preparations, deodorant soaps, antibiotics and antihistamines. They often create allergies, rashes and, occasionally, even infections. Avoid the sunburn preparations known as the "caines." They contain benzocaine and many people are allergic to it. In fact, benzocaine is so dangerous it is actually banned in some eastern European countries. There are at least four hundred products on the U.S. market that contain benzocaine.

Many anesthetics sold for sunburn and itchy skin actually develop skin reactions which produce blistering or poison ivy-type rash. These products contain antibacterial agents, causing users to become photosensitive so that, going out in the sun, they become severely burned. Rather than the "caine" sun products, use plain cold water or ice to treat all ordinary burns, including sunburn. And use aloe vera gel.

To correct a chapped and irritated face, apply a plain hot wet towel for five minutes, followed with a good moisturizer. Avoid using make-up as much as possible. To remove the dead cells and the old skin after a summer of suntanning, use a facial mask that contains an agent capable of peeling off the dead cells, such as Fanie's Mask. It will remove blackheads and whiteheads that may be lying directly under the skin. Finish with cleansing and an oily moisturizer.

To combat dryness from desert-like wind and air, steam the face at least once a week to restore moisture to your parched skin, then add this gel mask: to one package of lemon gelatin add lemon juice for half of the water required. Set in refrigerator until firm enough to coat the face as a mask. Let it remain ten minutes and remove with cool water.

Herbs

Herbs have been renowned not only for health but for cosmetic purposes since before biblical times. In these latter days they have fallen into disuse because of the advent of modern cosmetology and advertising persuasion. But now entering the market is a steady flow of not only health products but beauty cosmetics as well, derived directly from herbs and other plants, such as seaweed. Herbs are making a comeback, appearing on the world market in various forms. There are many which offer excellent benefits in cosmetics and facial rejuvenation.

Herbs may be used to deep cleanse, as a facial, as a night cream, as a moisturizer or as a shampoo. To use an herb for such purposes, prepare it as you usually make herb tea, but double the strength. Bring a cup of water to a rolling boil in a pan (not aluminum), remove from the stove, add a heaping tablespoon of herbs, cover, then allow it to steep 12 minutes, still covered. Strain and store in refrigerator. Fennel tea thus prepared is excellent to tighten skin and remove wrinkles. Apply it to skin with a pure cotton pat.

For a steam tea facial, deep cleansing or moisturizing, remove the steaming tea from the stove. As described earlier, bend your face directly over the steam, covering your head with a towel. Or use the herbal solution in your facial sauna. Finish the treatment with splashes of cold water, followed with a moisturizer. Or follow the steaming with a facial mask. Refrigerate the remaining tea to be patted on the face as a daily freshening lotion, or add it to your tub soak. Or prepare an herbal astringent lotion as follows:

In a wide mouth jar, place one pint of herb leaves — fennel is excellent. Cover them with apple cider vinegar, and place the lid tightly on the jar. Set the jar in a warm spot, preferably the direct sunlight, for two or even three weeks. Then strain through a fine strainer (steel). To a cup of the strained mixture add one cup of fresh cucumber juice and one teaspoon of benzoin tincture as a preservative (available from drug stores). Place this solution in a pan on the stove and bring to a boil. Pour it into a bottle and seal tightly. Keep this solution in your bathroom to be handily available as an astringent after each face wash or following face cleansing with a cream. This face tonic removes all traces of make-up, restores the acid balance to the skin, disinfects and moisturizes all at the same time. It also tightens the skin and removes wrinkles.

Certain herbs have been known and used to enhance intuition, insight and psychic faculties. In the days of antiquity — especially those of the Delphic Oracles of Greece — the virgins of the temples were renowned for their ability to discern the future for those seeking their intuitive and perceptive prophecies. They were reputed to use an herb called laurel. They slept on beds of laurel leaves, they chewed the laurel leaves, they drank laurel tea and laurel was an ingredient of the substance burned in a pit over which the oracle sat, perched atop a bronze tripod spanning the pit. The aroma and vapors of the herbal substance aided in her psychic state. Other psychic herbs include rosemary leaves, dried rose petals, comfrey, gotu kola, and fo-ti-tieng (fo-tee-ting), which is also supposed to aid longevity.

The Aloe Vera Plant — Ancient documents, written at least 3500 years ago, called the *Papyrus Ebers,* mention the miraculous virtues of aloe vera. The original papers are now found in Leipzig University. Armies of antiquity carried the leaves of the aloe vera cactus during their long marches. The gel was used to heal battle wounds and relieve untold skin problems. Alexander the Great made it a point to conquer the Island of Socotra in East Africa for the sole purpose of obtaining aloe vera as a medicinal agent to heal the wounds of his soldiers. Alexander was known to deploy his armies in the direction of lands where the precious plant might be found. All of the ancient Arabian caravans directed their routes where the cactus plant grew abundantly. There it was gathered and taken into far corners of the world. Biblical writings also may refer to aloe vera in the New Testament — John 19:39. This particular scripture describes the journey of Nicodemus who came by night with a mixture of myrrh and aloe to embalm the body of Jesus. It is believed that this aloe is the aloe vera plant often called Barbadensis.

Aloe vera is only now becoming recognized as a miracle plant in our day. I have heard a few reports that, mixed with drinking water and drunk daily, or applied to the skin (or both), cancers have been healed — not only skin cancers but those in the body. These claims may be exaggerated. I mention them only because those reporting these miracles were personally involved and spoke from personal experience. Aloe vera gel or juice could surely be added to any program of healing with beneficial results. Certainly aloe vera is recognized as beneficial for burn treatments, ulcer cures, acne, skin abrasions, boils, sunburn — and it is claimed that some of the Japanese population exposed to the A-bomb radiation applied aloe gel to their wounds. Those who did were cured far more rapidly than others, whereas thousands who did not use it were not cured at all.

Aloe has also been found to relieve itching skin, poison ivy, insect bites and stings, to heal eczema and the *agony of shingles*.

The best method of cleansing a wound is simply to wash it in mild soap and water. Avoid painting it with iodine or putting antibiotics on it. Iodine is much too strong. Antibiotic ointments often prove far more harmful than good, resulting in serious infections. Instead, apply aloe vera gel.

I add from two to four ounces of aloe vera gel to my morning orange juice, along with all the other ingredients I'll mention. It adds enzymes to the digestive system; it oxygenizes the cells; it improves the memory. I use it, too, on my face and throat and the rejuvenating effect is obvious. When taking Hanna Kroeger's *Circu-Flow* herbal capsules to clear out hardened arteries (oral chelation), she instructs they be taken with aloe vera gel because she knows aloe vera aids the process. Its benefits seem endless.

When I was writing *The Book of Beginning Again,* I contacted the late Betty Lee Morales, a renowned writer and lecturer for health organizations, and a very dear friend. I asked for any kind of contribution in writing I might use in that book. She finally submitted an article but it did not arrive until after the book was being printed. So I'm using her article now. It's important. Betty chose aloe vera to write about. Here is the article she forwarded:

"Miracle herbs and cure-alls form the centralized factor-fiction core of lore the world around, and it would require a blasé soul indeed to gainsay the claims made for any one of them.

"Natives and old-timers, wherever man's feet have trod, tell tales of wondrous 'cures' and life-saving properties of roots and herbs, of flower essences, of barks and berries, and about everything else in Nature's domain. It seems that everywhere Nature has provided aid and comfort for human beings, as well as for the animals and birds who know instinctively where to seek their 'medicine,' and when. Man has not generally been so intuitive, since his primeval evolvement, and more particularly since the popularity of the broad spectrum antibiotics and the time-saving 'shots' of antihistamines, synthetic hormones and serums. It is refreshing, and a sort of validation to those favoring nature-cure, to contemplate the virtues of a real 'wonder plant,' often spoken of by natives as 'the medicine plant,' or 'Heaven's Blessing.'

"This, of course, could be none other than the aloe, which is known to have over 200 different types or species! The one most widely used by natives the world over, wherever it is indigenous to the region, is the one called aloe vera. Aloe vera looks like a member of the cactus family, and closely resembles the Century Plant, with its tall spear-like growth and saw-tooth edges. But don't let looks steer you in the wrong direction, for aloe vera is really a lily, as is the onion, another cousin. Lost in antiquity is the history of the discovery of the virtues of the aloe, but legend tells us that the Mayan maidens, famed for velvety skin and luxuriant gleaming hair, claimed aloe vera as their gift from Venus, the Goddess of Love.

"While I was studying years ago at the University of Mexico, in Mexico City, one of the professors of biochemistry remarked that the Mexican Indians were almost never bald and seldom gray. He claimed it was because they habitually rubbed the thick, gelatinous juice from the aloe vera leaves well into the scalp and hair, allowing it to remain on overnight, prior to washing. Upon application as directed the gooey, gelatinous mass (or mess) gave rise to wonder, but miracle of miracles, it was absorbed into the hair and scalp within a few hours, and left the hair with the appearance of having been heavily oiled. However, upon shampooing, no soap or shampoo was needed as the aloe vera foamed better than any commercial product. What's more, no cream rinse or other concoction of the cosmetic geniuses of Hollywood and Paris could have left the hair so clean — actually squeaky clean — or so shiny and manageable.

"Limitation of supply prevented an objective evaluation of the actual long-range improvement in hair quality or color resulting from the use of aloe vera, but as a dressing or shampoo one application is sufficient to make a lasting impression.

"While visiting David ('Daddy') Bray, on the Kona side of the Big Island of Hawaii, and walking through his charming grounds and gardens, we again learned of the virtues of aloe vera, lovingly called 'Alloy' by most Hawaiians. (Note from Earlyne — 'Daddy' Bray was a renowned Hawaiian Kahuna. He lectured many times at our church and shared many healing 'secrets' with Dr. Robert and me.) Snipping off a young aloe vera plant shoot and breaking it in two to allow the gelatinous fluid to ooze out, 'Daddy' remarked, 'Why don't you rub this on your sunburn? Here, try it on the back of your neck, which will surely blister and peel if you don't.'

"The first contact of the fluid with the too-hot skin was like a cool blessing, a veritable benediction. The sting and fiery hurt melted away and the skin fairly gulped the soothing jelly-liquid as soon as it hit the surface. Sticky at first, within a minute or two the skin was smooth and dry, and remarkably comfortable. Another score for aloe! And just as David Bray promised, the skin did not blister or peel.

"What the fashion magazines don't tell about aloe is that its healing juices are just as beneficial to the insides of man as they are to the outside. Mexicans and Indians in our hemisphere have long used the juice, which is more like a gel after extraction, as a tonic for better digestion, and for relief of ulcers and poor elimination. In itself not laxative or only mildly so, the aloe is believed to improve digestion and assimilation of food eaten, so that elimination is naturally normalized. This concept is in accordance with the Chinese or oriental philosophy of medicine, and goes back more than 5000 years in their recorded history.

"True nature enthusiasts should value the aloe vera in as near a natural state as possible, unpasteurized and free of preservatives. How better to secure a continuing supply of this wonder herb than to cultivate a plant or two? It's decorative, hardy, virtually pest-free and surely the most versatile plant that grows!" So said Betty Lee Morales.

Eyes That Are Puffy — especially in the morning, could suggest retained fluid which, in turn, indicates a sluggish kidney-bladder functioning. Buchu herb capsules, watermelon seed tea or capsules, or cranberry juice or capsules, could be an excellent internal treatment. An external treatment is, again, to splash the eyes with water. Alternately splash with cold, then hot, then cold water, finishing with cold. Also apply Dr. Christopher's Eyebright herbal tea solution to each eye with a cotton pat and relax a few minutes. Cucumber slices over your eyes will reduce puffiness. It will also, through osmosis, aid in getting "the red" out and remove blurring.

Chapter Four

Healing Skin Problems

Fungus Infections — Fungus infections are a common cause for skin problems, the most common being ringworm. A ringworm infection can become inflamed, itchy and scaly. It often erupts on the feet as athlete's foot, but sometimes it appears on the back of the neck or elsewhere on the back of the head, on the nails and in the groin. There are several over-the-counter medications which have proven effective such as *Undecyleinic Acid* or *Tolnaftate*. For athlete's foot, always dry the feet thoroughly after a bath. Apply a good foot powder and cover with cotton or wool socks. Avoid wearing sneakers which tend to aggravate a fungus infection. Sneakers are also reputed to cause cancer. More about this in *The You Book*.

Itchy Skin — There are ten foods which sometimes cause an itchy skin rash, especially in children. The leading culprits are eggs, peanuts and pasteurized milk. Should your child be allergic to milk, do seek for raw milk before you give up. If eggs, try eggs from a health store from chickens with barnyard freedom. The other foods are wheat, soy products, chicken, pork, beef, fish and potatoes. Almost all children tend to outgrow these youth allergies after a couple of years, but some allergies remain throughout a lifetime. If your child suffers from a bumpy, itchy skin rash and the doctor has not been able to pinpoint the problem, do try eliminating these allergy foods to see if there's an improvement. Then return one at a time to the diet, to discover which food to blame or if the allergy has been outgrown.

If there are continuing problems, try eliminating the nightshade foods which include potatoes, tomatoes, peppers, and all tobacco products. If the skin problem persists, see an allergy specialist for eliminating other common allergy foods. A hair analysis may be considered, especially if dizziness is present. A hair analysis would indicate whether heavy metal toxicity is present. Do check also for chemical exposure, such as slow leaking natural gas, exposure to asbestos or exposure to formaldehyde.

Skin Cancer — Although it usually is not fatal, about 6,000 people die each year from neglected skin cancer. See a doctor immediately if you have a mole, wart or pigmented area that appears suddenly, starts to grow, bleed or change color. Or if you have a sore that is persistent. Ninety-eight percent of skin cancers can usually be cured by a single treatment, such as surgical excision, or freezing with liquid nitrogen. Malignant melanoma is the most dangerous skin disease. It affects about 14,000 Americans each year and kills about 4,300. Fair-skinned people are subject to this malignancy which appears as a flat or slightly raised brown or black spot that looks like an ordinary mole. Do see a doctor immediately because such a melanoma can spread quickly.

Sun exposure is the major cause. The Fanie distributors

listed in the last chapter declare skin lesions to have been healed by using their Oak Bark Skin Cleanser followed by Fanie's Herbal Oils. Contact Karie Hayden or Carlis Orlando for full information and guidance (last chapter). Fanie offers other products which have been known to prevent skin lesions.

Dr. Norman Brooks of the University of California at Los Angeles reports a new technique for banishing skin cancer without leaving scars. It's called Mohs micrographic surgery, which involves shaving thin layers from the skin until no evidence of the cancer remains. Each layer is tested for tumor cells as it's removed. Such a treatment should improve the entire face since all the dead cells would also be removed. See *The You Book: A Treasury of Health and Healing* for information regarding removing skin cancer with garlic poultices.

For Bloodshot Eyes — Lean over the wash basin and splash the eyes with cold water many times. The water will act as a blood vessel constrictor, shrinking the capillaries. Avoid using products from the drug store which promise to "get the red out." They often cause deeper irritation. The only drug store product I recommend for an eyewash is *Lavoptic*, which not only aids in clearing away the bloodshot condition, but will remove strands of mucus which often form under the eyelids. Preferably, choose an eyewash from health stores. Ask for *Similasan* Eye Drops, a homeopathic remedy. Or *Katalyse* drops, excellent for cataracts or inflammation. Order from Hanna Kroeger. Or choose an herbal solution of eyebright tea — obviously effective because of its name. Dr. John Christopher produces an *Eyebright* herbal capsule which has proven excellent for the eyes. You empty the capsule contents into a cup, add hot water, steep it for at least six minutes, strain it and wash the eyes in the cooled herbal solution. The longer it's steeped, the better. Be sure to use a glass eye cup, not plastic. And be sure to use a steel strainer, not aluminum. Make fresh tea every third day. Drink any remaining tea. Other herbal teas of benefit to eyes include verbena, fennel or elderflower.

Vertical Lip Lines — When deep vertical lines appear on the upper lip it often indicates a lack of vitamin B. Try brewer's yeast tablets. Or Fanie's liquid vitamin B under the tongue. Also try this facial exercise: Open the lips and draw them taut over the teeth in a wide smile. Then massage the upper lip vigorously with a horizontal stroke, rubbing opposite the wrinkles, as if attempting to erase them. Apply an oil or moisturizer to the lip or fingertip for the massage. The lines should soon fade. In Chapter One, see Sanford Bennett's facial exercise for removing these wrinkles. Also see my own suggestion of massaging upon awakening after applying Beleza cream to the upper lip.

Stress — can trigger psoriasis, shingles, eczema, vitiligo, and even cold sores. Even positive events such as vacations can cause stress. I always found vacations very stressful — car trouble, lost baggage, cold hotels, hot hotels, soft mattresses, hard mattresses, noisy early morning departures, screaming children in the room next door, a lost driver who is reluctant to seek directions at a service station. Anyway, as Robert always says, to have a fun vacation you have to work at it, and "make it an adventure." He's learned to "stay cool" under all circumstances, while I run around climbing walls. To stay cool no matter what or where, is the point. But do be aware that your emotions affect your skin. *The You Book: A Treasury of Health and Healing* contains much about certain supplements which alleviate stress and build the immune system to cope. It seems redundant to repeat it here. But I do want to mention Fanie's sublingual (under the tongue) vitamin B complex which is excellent for stress. Or seek herbal solutions for relaxing tensions rather than tranquilizers. Contact Hanna Kroeger or Michael Tierra for herbal suggestions for emotional as well as physical problems. (See last chapter.)

Treating and Removing Skin Blemishes

Birthmarks — There's a new painless laser treatment reputed to "fade-out" unsightly birthmarks. Do seek the advice of a good dermatologist. Or try Fanie's Herbal Oil.

Blemishes — Apply a Q-Tip dipped in witch hazel to a pimple to dry it up, or dab on Calamine Lotion. It should vanquish the pimple overnight. Enrich your night cream with a teaspoon of liquid vitamin C and vitamin E. I must mention, too, *Fanie's Blemish Gel* which is simply marvelous for treating all manner of skin blemishes.

Boils — A friend writes to say that she removed a boil by applying mashed figs as a poultice. If you have a stubborn boil that refuses to heal, you may wish to try it. Do consult your doctor first. Or try Fanie's Blemish Gel. Its deep down heating action is extremely effective for treating boils.

Brown Spots — or yellowing of the skin may indicate a liver problem or a lack of fluoride, which should be obtained through a natural mineral tablet, never through drinking water. The mineral tablet would contain *all* the natural minerals, blended by God, not man. Or consider *Fanie's Brown Spot Oil* or Retinol-A for vanquishing brown spots. A patch test is suggested for possible allergic reaction.

Cold Sores, Fever Blisters and Herpes Virus — The best abortive product I've found is *Neosporin*. Second, *Campho-Phenique*. Apply generously and often. Also, surprise! t ry ice cubes. Try milk which has been removed from the refrigerator for at least fifteen minutes. Try a squeezed out tea bag directly over the sore. Eat yogurt as a preventive. Or try Fanie's Blemish Gel. Its deep heat therapy burns out infections. I think you begin to understand that the Fanie products are far more than a "cosmetic" or beauty product — they are carefully formulated skin treatments not only for beauty but for all skin problems.

Cysts — These are usually removed by a doctor with a scalpel.

Eczema — Add PABA, or para-aminobenzoic acid, to the diet. And try Fanie's *Procaine Cream*. It's great. Procaine differs totally from the "caines" mentioned earlier. However, it would be well to consider a skin test.

Moles — Most doctors remove moles by shaving them off with a scalpel. Larger ones must be cut out and the area closed with stitches. Shortly afterward the skin heals completely. You may want to try Fanie's Herbal Oil before seeking scalpel removal. Persistent use has been known to eventually remove moles and other blemishes.

Spider Veins — A solution which seals the blood vessels and causes them to disappear is injected directly into the veins by a dermatologist.

Warts — Warts on the hands and fingers are usually painless and go away without treatment. Generally within six months to a year. On the soles of the feet warts are called planter warts and are often painful. Try castor oil, applied every night and morning until the wart disappears. Or apply Fanie's *Thymolize* or Herbal Oil. Or ask your doctor to prescribe a homeopathic remedy called

Tumorel and drop the prescribed drops under your tongue. In a few days the wart should fall off, no matter where it is on the body. I know a lady who removed a wart from her foot using this remedy under the tongue. Or see a podiatrist who will remove it with liquid nitrogen or surgery. Nitrogen freezes the tissue and disintegrates the wart.

Another remedy is to soak a dab of cotton with apple cider vinegar and apply it to the wart with a Band-Aid or other adhesive. Apply the vinegar only occasionally for three days. It may be advisable to apply after working hours and at bedtime since it may be difficult to keep it on during daily activities. The wart should disappear, never to return. If applied too abundantly you may experience a slight burning sensation from the vinegar reaching the live root too quickly.

Dry Skin, Arthritis and Psoriasis

Dry skin, when all is said and done, must be cured interiorly. Exterior creams will not wholly eliminate the problem. Moisturizers will certainly moisturize the skin as long as they are used but once one ceases to use them, the dry skin returns so, obviously, moisturizers cannot effect a total cure. A new layer of outer skin is born every twenty-seven days.

Can there possibly be a connection between dry skin and arthritis? — and psoriasis? Just as Dale Alexander made cod liver oil popular for arthritic sufferers, he maintains it simultaneously lubricates the skin and keeps it moist. Cod liver oil contains vitamin A, excellent for the skin, vitamin D which is important for strong bones, phosphorus needed for tissue repair, and essential fatty acids, which heal skin blemishes. Dale maintains that this interior lubricant not only heals arthritis but also removes dryness of the skin and dryness of the scalp. *He suggests that drinking water with meals invariably results in some form of dry skin and dry joints.* I heartily agree. It also results in poor digestion, especially if the water is iced. He says — and I agree — that drinking water with meals affects the way oils are absorbed. That's because oil and water do not mix, which is common knowledge. Thus the oil released by the food cannot mix with the water ingested at the same time and prevents the oil from lubricating all the systems in the body. For the natural oils in the food to lubricate and heal the skin and joints, it must bypass the liver. If it does not, the liver captures the oils and uses them to produce fat. When you drink water with meals the liver gets most of the oils and the skin suffers. And the joints get dry. And arthritis and dry skin are the result. And perhaps even baldness, because of a dry scalp.

According to Dale Alexander, if you have dry skin, you have much more than dry skin. You have dryness throughout the body, which means the joints need lubricating. Your hair, eyes, ears, nerves, muscles, blood vessels and even the blood cells need lubricating. When your skin is dry, your hair and scalp are also dry. Your skin itches, your scalp itches, your ears itch, and the joints in your body "squeak" when you stoop or bend. You also probably have no ear wax, and loss of ear wax is often followed by ringing in the ears, then hearing loss and often deafness. So, it would behoove us to think in terms of cod liver oil, or some other Omega 3 natural oil, such as flaxseed oil.

Dale Alexander says: One hour before breakfast, take one tablespoon of the cod liver oil every morning with two ounces of whole raw milk shaken together until it foams. You may prefer two ounces of fresh strained orange juice but the oil is much more effective when mixed with milk. Take cod liver oil capsules, if you prefer, but they aren't as effective. When you notice that the dryness of the hair or scalp seems to be corrected, taper down slowly on your oil-milk shake. Take it every other morning for approximately six months. Then taper off to once a week. He claims it also heals arthritis.

Those who have gall bladder problems, or have had it removed, should use only a teaspoon of cod liver oil on alternate days. And those with high blood pressure, heart disease or diabetes should take it every other night or twice a week. Those with eczema, psoriasis, dermatitis, any type of ulcer or skin irritation owing to nerve involvement, should mix the oil only with whole milk because those with the above ailments are often allergic to the citric acid of oranges. I have never tried the oil-milk treatment myself, but it has received wide acceptance, especially in combating arthritis, for which it is renowned. You might wish to try it, with your doctor's consent, of course. Also, if you have tinnitus — ringing in the ears.

Psoriasis — At least a million Americans suffer from this persistent, recurring, disfiguring disease. Doctors claim it is inherited, but it is the result of excessive secretions of oil from the sebaceous glands which block the ducts conducting oil to the surface of the skin, as in acne. It's called sebum. Psoriasis usually begins between the teen years and the thirties, commonly appearing on the knees, fingernails, elbows, and the scalp. It is recognized by itchy red plaque often covered with a silvery scale that peels off like sheets of mica. Doctors claim there is no cure but there are many effective treatments. Regular exposure to the sun is suggested, but be cautious. Often an ointment that contains corticosteroids is recommended, but only as a last resort. Consider giving up homogenized milk, which could be a cause. Switch to raw whole certified milk. If unavailable, try eliminating milk entirely and see what happens. Use raw sweet butter, not homogenized salted. Riboflavin and unsaturated fats should be added to the diet. Vitamin D3 ointment is now being used successfully to treat psoriasis.

I must tell you about Clyde Johnson's (Fanie) special formula for treating psoriasis or shingles. It's so "special" that, prior to his death, sufferers from around the world contacted him for help. Each client was treated individually — that is, he discussed each client's problem personally, then formulated a treatment cream especially for that person. If you have a problem with psoriasis or shingles, you may wish to contact Karie Hayden, R.C., or Carlis Orlando, R.C., estheticians-educators for Fanie, via telephone for a personal consultation. The cream is totally "natural," made exclusively from herbs. Both Karie and Carlis have been trained for years by both Florence and Clyde Johnson.

Or you may want to try the cod liver oil-milk drink suggested earlier, or Omega 3 capsules, or flaxseed oil. Speaking of the oil and psoriasis, researchers in England have proven fish oil heals this dreadful inflammation of the skin. They gave psoriasis patients ten fish oil capsules a day and instructed them to continue eating their customary diet. The report did not say what kind of fish oil capsules were used. Possibly cod liver oil. The symptoms began to disappear after eight weeks. The itching, redness and scaling dramatically improved. If you suffer with psoriasis, you may wish to try it. Or you may wish to substitute the fish oil for flaxseed oil. Perhaps such a test would also prove beneficial for arthritics. Eat a lot of sunflower seeds which contain natural vitamins A and B. Use olive or sesame oil in the kitchen. Also contact Hanna Kroeger and Michael Tierra for herbal products which could heal the inflammation.

Good news concerns a prescription drug called *Anthralin*. It's reported to be extremely effective. High doses rubbed on the skin, left on for ten minutes, then washed off, are as effective as the lower dose applied for three or four hours. The high dose also causes less redness and itching in removing psoriasis scales.

A new lotion can bring fast relief to scalp psoriasis. It's called *Diprolene Lotion*. It also works rapidly against seborrheic dermatitis, which causes a dry or greasy scaling on the scalp. Diprolene Lotion contains a steroid called bethamethasone diproprionate, so you'll need a prescription. It should be treated by a dermatologist.

Thousands with psoriasis flock to bathe in the waters of the Dead Sea near Israel. Its mysterious contents give miraculous relief to the painful symptoms. Dead Sea salts are now available at many health stores for use in tub soaks. Do try it for any kind of skin ailment.

A skin patch called *Actiderm* is now being used to treat psoriasis. It works most often in conjunction with the most common psoriasis medication-steroid ointments. It isn't a cure, but it does make the affliction more comfortable. There's also a home treatment available, an anticancer drug called *5-Fluorouracil*, better known as *5-FU*. It's rubbed on the problem area once a week, then covered with a plastic wrap for 24 hours. Do ask your doctor about it if you're afflicted. I've suggested several drug-chemical treatments, but keep in mind that Fanie's formula is totally from herbs.

Flaxseed Oil — may be preferred over cod liver oil. Many may prefer the flaxseed oil simply because it's a plant derivative. It's rich in Omega 3, which is also excellent for heart problems. Flaxseed oil probably would be just as effective for arthritis or any of the other complaints as cod liver oil, and is now being offered in palatable form at every health store, or order from Swanson's Health Catalog (address in Chapter 10). If you have arthritis, psoriasis or dry skin, do try either of the oils. You may find your arthritis healed, plus a radiant new skin. Youth and beauty from within. I add a tablespoon of Spectrum Naturals Flaxseed Oil to my orange juice breakfast drink. I also add a teaspoon each of brewer's yeast flakes, lecithin granules, goat milk whey, chlorophyll, and a teaspoon of Vitality Food (mixed seeds and dried fruits), all available from National Fruit and Vegetables Industries (address in Chapter 10). I also add a dash of aloe vera gel. With this drink, I eat five fresh-shelled almonds.

Shingles — At last there seems to be a product that offers relief from the agony of shingles. It's called *Zostrix*. You'll need a doctor's prescription. Reports state it will almost immediately relieve pain and itching. It's a cream that is easily applied. Another new medicated cream is called *Genderm*. Both Zostrix and GenDerm are creams containing a substance known as capsaicin, which is the active ingredient in red peppers. Also experiment with taking *cayenne* herbal capsules made from red peppers, available at your health store. Cayenne is also excellent to increase blood circulation. Also antidepressant drugs are proving effective as excellent pain relievers of shingles,

But if you'd like to stay away from prescription drugs, I refer you again to Fanie's special treatment cream especially for your shingles problem. You may wish to order the regular cream for shingles, or call Karie Hayden or Carlis Orlando personally so that either may create your own individualized formula.

Acne and Other Skin Problems — Let's speak first of acne. Acne normally occurs during the teen years. It's usually caused by a hormonal imbalance which causes an increase in oil secreting glands (sebaceous glands) of the face, shoulders and arms. Puberty is a time when hormones are becoming active through the development of the endocrine glands. These hormones often force the sebaceous glands into overactivity, creating an excessive oil in the skin. The oil, traveling through the pores, mixes with surface dirt. The glands often become plugged with oil and debris, forming blackheads, whiteheads, and cysts. Pimples result when they become infected.

However, acne is now appearing not only among teens but among women aged 25 to 45. These career woman are experiencing acne due to stress, the use of cosmetics containing allergy-related substances, the birth control pill and various environmental pollutants. The cosmetics causing the increase in acne are cleansing creams, night moisturizers, face foundations, and rouges that contain derivatives of coal tar products and oils and derivatives of fatty acids. Vitamin supplements sometimes contribute because they contain too much iodine.

The diet is also involved. Research confirms that the diet of those with acne and other skin problems invariably points to foods that rob them of B vitamins and vitamin C. Many acne sufferers seem to prefer foods and drinks from which these essentials have been eliminated by processing. The presence of acne, psoriasis, or any other skin problem indicates a lack of vitamin B6, vitamin D, and biotin. Niacin and B-Complex vitamin supplements often help relieve itching skin problems. Try massaging with cold pressed castor oil. Also try aloe vera gel.

Certain foods seem to increase an acne problem. These include chocolate, iodized salt, cola drinks, fried food, shell-fish and some nuts, especially if they are roasted and salt-ed. Such skin afflictions also indicate an adrenal deficien-cy. Licorice herb capsules have been known to stimulate the adrenals, but don't overdo. Licorice can cause heart problems. Also lobelia and ginger stimulate the adrenals.

May I share with you the results of my own research concerning acne:

1. It's obvious that the skin must be kept meticulously clean from any dirt particles which might mix with the excessive oils. But it must be observed that the diet should be low in undesirable carbohydrates and fats. Do try mas-sive doses of vitamin A for a short time to discover the effect. It usually has a remarkably healing effect because it balances the flow of the oil in the skin. Don't stay on a massive intake of vitamin A. It can be toxic. It would be wise, when one enters the age of puberty, to begin small regular doses of vitamin A. Such a plan might prevent acne from happening at all.

2. Dr. C. Ralph Campo of the University of Psychic Science in Lemon Grove, California, states that *roquefort* cheese can help clear up acne as well as other ailments, because it contains natural penicillin. "Pimples, boils and tumors simply disappear." He says many people swear that it helps their digestion, cures ulcers and relieves asthma and other respiratory problems. He suggests placing a small piece of the cheese under the tongue immediately after waking and just before bedtime. This "homeopathic" approach enables the penicillin to more directly enter the bloodstream.

3. Some people are sensitive to woolen clothing, others to synthetic fabrics. Switch to cotton. Cotton clothing is readily available today and is much more comfortable then synthetic products or fabrics produced from the animal kingdom

4. *Retinoic acid* is occasionally prescribed to be taken orally. It should never be taken except under the supervision of a doctor acquainted with its use. Side effects have been known to occur. It should never be taken during pregnancy — it has been known to cause fetal abnormalities. Retinoic acid (Retin-A) may also be applied topically to the acne after carefully cleansing the skin. Again, when used for acne, Retin-A (vitamin A) should only be applied under the direction of a physician, preferably a dermatologist.

However, scientists have developed a new form of vitamin A that can be used without risky side effects. It is combined with a sugar-like substance which makes it water soluble and easily absorbed by the body. The new compound will be used for treating not only acne, but psoriasis and wrinkling, as well. Ask your doctor about it.

5. Instead of an over-the-counter acne medication, try *Sul-Ray Acne Treatment Cream* from your health store. If unavailable ask the store to order from Alvin Last, Inc. Or write directly to the address given in the last chapter. It contains natural ingredients, especially sulfur, a natural antidote to infection. Discuss its use with your dermatologist.

6. Many turn to *benzoyl peroxide*, an over-the-counter product, and use it once or twice a day. Avoid all such products, if possible. They may be filled with synthetic properties dangerous to the bloodstream. If you feel you must use it, start with a 5% solution. If that does not appear to

be successful, try a 10% solution, if your doctor agrees.

7. Always apply ice to the skin for five minutes twice a day before applying the acne medication. It aids in healing the acne. The cold encourages slight peeling of the skin so helps the medication to penetrate. If your medication is benzoyl peroxide, the ice treatment boosts its effectiveness.

8. Do keep your hair well off your face. Oily hair is dangerous. Shampoo the hair often. Wash your face with a very mild chemical-free and natural cleansing lotion (perhaps Fanie's Oak Bark Cleanser) and lukewarm water twice daily. Use tepid water. Use a very clean washcloth. Do not rub vigorously. Rub gently. If you choose Fanie's Cleanser then you may not want to use a cloth at all — just splash over the face and gently massage with your hands.

9. Do consider ceasing birth control pills. They sometimes cause acne. Try the diaphragm, plus an over-the-counter vaginal suppository for double protection. Remember, there are only five days out of the month you are fertile for impregnation. Why not learn the rhythm system to discover which days?

10. When shopping for a make-up base, consider one with a matte finish to avoid oil on your face. Choose hypoallergenic cosmetics, such as Physician's Formula, available at drug stores. Or Creative Illusions liquid cream foundation which is oil-free and marvelous. (Address elsewhere). Avoid astringents and products with alcohol. Most of them stimulate the oil glands. Use a moisturizer with vitamin E, which is a great aid to troubled skin.

11. Products to be avoided are those that contain lanolin, isopropyl, myristate or derivatives, and detergents such as sodium lauryl sulfate or laurath-4. Stay away also

from any products containing D and C red colors on the label. Many blushers contain bright reds and should be avoided. Use a red eye shadow for a blusher until acne is cured, after consulting your dermatologist. Or shop at a health store for a blusher with natural contents, such as *Aubrey Organics*. Do not take a multivitamin containing iodine or iodide.

12. Avoid "picking" at your face. Is it possible just squeezing a pimple could kill you? Indeed it could, if the blemish is in the area between the eyebrows and extending down to the corners of the mouth — and this is where most pimples and blackheads flourish. Blood vessels link this area directly to the brain. If the squeezed pimple or blackhead contracts a bacterial infection, the bacteria could enter the bloodstream through the broken skin and rush to the brain, causing permanent damage or even death. Thus all squeezing and picking at blemishes in this area should be avoided. Even if it does not lead to serious infection, squeezing pimples may cause permanent scars.

13. *Accutane*, used only for severe cases of acne, is a derivative of vitamin A. It has proven effective in about 90% of cystic-acne patients. It has also reduced the development of skin cancer. But it can't be widely used. It contains substances which have serious side effects in some patients. It can't be given pregnant women because it can cause birth defects. It also causes liver problems and raises the level of cholesterol.

14. *Isotretinoin* capsule is also a vitamin A derivative developed to heal stubborn and severe cystic-acne. Side effects include drying of lips, joint pain, muscle aches, and changes in blood lipid levels. However, only a small percentage experience these side effects. Your doctor may try it cautiously.

15. *Tetracycline*, an oral antibiotic, is often prescribed, but do try other methods first because tetracycline has dreadful side effects, as well as often resulting in vaginal yeast infection. Do ask your doctor to relate the side effects before embarking on this antibiotic approach. Topical antibiotics are applied directly on the site of the acne.

16. Do write to Karie Hayden or Carlis Orlando concerning Fanie's excellent treatment for acne. Fanie offers time-proven products to heal and subdue this problem. If you live in the Southern California area, do consider contacting Karie Hayden or Carlis Orlando's Center for a special facial treatment. You'll find trained cosmetologists there who will use special therapies to correct your individual problem. Based on Clyde Johnson's Fanie Products, either of them will create your own individual formula. If you live elsewhere, call or write Fanie for a treatment salon in your area. They are nationwide. (See last chapter for address).

17. The National Cancer Institute in Washington has released a report stating that over a million Americans who received radiation treatments for acne during their teens should be tested for possible thyroid cancer. It requires from five to forty-five years for radiation-caused thyroid cancer to develop. Do check your throat for lumps in the thyroid if you were treated with radiation. They would appear at the base of the throat on either side of the Adam's apple.

18. The FDA has recently approved a drug called *Metrogel* which was developed especially for adult acne and will soon be on the market. I have no firsthand knowledge of it, but perhaps it will prove beneficial to some.

Acne Scars — Frequently the skin is "sanded down" through a process called dermabrasion. Another treatment injects collagen into soft depressions to eliminate the depression. Four or five sessions may be necessary, with a follow-up in a year or so. Deeper "ice pick" scars may require a combination of dermabrasion and surgical removal. Retin-A is now being tried and is proving effective in removing scars. Strong vitamin E oil applied topically on the site of the blemish has worked marvels. Buy it at your health store. Or write *Genesis West* to inquire if their live cell therapy would help acne scars. Dr. Robert Harmon's skin peel mentioned earlier would probably be very effective, or the laser treatment at the Hermosa Beach clinic. (See last chapter).

Tell-Tale Signs of Health

The skin is a mouthpiece for health, giving ample warnings of approaching problems. Here are some signs it displays:

1. Sudden itching of the feet and lower legs accompanied by burning may indicate Hodgkin's disease.

2. If a spot develops that looks like a target — a ring within a ring — it may indicate herpes infection or internal malignancy.

3. Jaundice or red spidery-like blood vessels on the surface of the skin could indicate trouble in the liver.

4. Broken blood vessels: cirrhosis of the liver.

5. Coin-sized, gray-blue areas on the trunk of the body could indicate leukemia.

6. An area of little black and blue spots all over the body could indicate malignancy. Or the need for vitamin C.

7. A raised bump with a pearly border and a little red line on the border could indicate a skin cancer.

8. Little bumps around the eyelids often indicate lipoproteinemia, which increases the possibility of a heart attack or diabetes.

9. Yellow spots around the eyelids may indicate fatty tumors in the body.

10. A cobblestone appearance of the skin on the front of the legs could mean too much thyroid hormone.

11. A firm yellow shiny depressed patch on the front of your shin almost always indicates diabetes.

12. Eczema on the palms of the hands or bottoms of the feet, caused by a certain type of sweating, could indicate an ulcer. Avoid wearing sneakers, which could cause cancer. Again, see *The You Book* for full information.

13. A slate-gray or blue-black fingernail could indicate silver or lead poisoning. (Silver dental fillings?) Green nails may indicate exposure to chrome. Blue nails to cobalt. A totally white nail, a serious liver condition. A nail that is half white and half red: kidney disease.

14. Sudden appearance of thirty or forty brown spots on the back and chest: internal malignancy, possibly cancer of the lungs.

15. Nodule on the tip of a finger, or on your eartips: gout.

16. Swollen ankles: kidney problems.

17. Big red scaly patches that won't go away: internal cancer.

18. Velvety rash under the arms, at the corners of your mouth, on the neck, or around the tongue: internal cancer such as the colon or ovaries.

19. Red butterfly-shaped rash across the nose and cheeks: lupus, a progressive type of inflammation affecting the skin, the joints and internal organs. (See *The You Book.*)

20. Change in a mole or wart: skin cancer.

21. Varicose veins: liver problems.

Chapter Five

Cosmetics

The common ingredients of many cosmetics are: beeswax, carnauba wax, candelilla wax, osokerite wax, castor oil, mineral oil, propylene glycol, glycerin, myristyl lactate, sodium laurel sulfate, magnesium aluminum silicate, talc, etc., etc., on and on, ad infinitum. Some add propylparaben, which can cause allergic reaction to sensitive skins. It's almost impossible to find cosmetics that don't contain at least some of these ingredients. I've tried to select those that contain the *least* objectionable. Apparently, cosmetics can't be manufactured without using some of these.

Be aware that the cosmetics you use could actually trigger an allergy attack. Certain ingredients cause itching and irritation — some can even cause acne. Test yours. If you have a dripping nose or itchy skin or eyes shortly after applying your make-up, test each item you use to discover which could be causing your problem — your base, powder, rouge, mascara? When you discover the culprit, switch brands until you find the brand which is harmless to your sensitive skin or eyes.

The test: choose an at-home day. Apply first your moisturizer. Wait a few moments. If your nose begins to drip or your skin itch, you're allergic. If no dripping, apply next your make-up base. Wait. Apply next your powder and wait. If, after one of the items you use, your nose begins to drip, you've found the culprit. Discard it and switch brands. If there is no dripping, you aren't allergic to your make-up. If the eyes itch, switch mascaras. I had to stop using Physician's Formula even though it's hypoallergenic. I now use Creative Illusions mascara.

Masks or Scrubs — Many contain the basics of water, oil, wax, powder and some sort of abrasive. Many people have serious reactions to "home" remedies, such as oatmeal, almond meal, or ground nuts. Choose a mask or scrub carefully. Some can actually damage your skin because they irritate too deeply. Avoid the use of any mask or scrub if your skin remains red or itchy even after removing.

Moisturizers — always contain water. Many add waxes and fats to stabilize the water, such as petrolatum (Vaseline) and mineral oil — very undesirable unless fractured. Often a paraben will be added as a preservative — you could be allergic. And, again, avoid glycerin. Do test any moisturizer which contains: isopropyl palmitate, parabens, glycerin, isopropyl myristate, mineral oil, cocoa butter, linseed oil, acetylated lanolin alcohol. It seems impossible to find a moisturizer without some of these. But you *can* choose one which contains the least. Of course, most people are not allergic to *any* of these. If you are, there's always the juice of cucumber. You may want to try Beleza's Anti-Aging Cream as a totally natural night moisturizer. Its honey-enzyme contents make it an excellent choice for the upward-stroke massage. And Patricia Allison's totally natural Vita Balm under your make-up as a daytime moisturizer. They both contain marvelous skin nourishers. Fanie's have far too many excellent choices to mention here, one for every skin type — all with herbs, moisture, and good things. See the last chapter for information about their many choices of moisturizers. *Suma*, by Jason, available in health stores, is excellent.

Anti-Aging — Beleza's Anti-Aging Cream, as just stated, is an excellent night moisturizer and skin rejuvenator. Beleza also offers a lotion to be used before your make-up base which does wonders. Patricia Allison has a white lotion to be used before your make-up base which makes lines temporarily disappear. It's used on top of her Vita Balm and it's followed by her make-up base. Most of Fanie's creams are anti-aging, especially her Fine Line Cream.

Astringents, Fresheners — most contain water, alcohol and/or witch hazel, all used for the purpose of absorbing oil. Some add zinc or aluminum to further remove oil. These should be avoided. The above ingredients can cause extreme irritation. Also avoid if their ingredients include menthol or camphor. Some contain lemon, eucalyptus or mint, which could benefit your skin unless it is extremely sensitive. Again, Patricia Allison offers a Wild Fern Freshener which is totally natural. Both of Fanie's Cleansers are natural astringents since they contain white oak bark, so you don't need an astringent or freshener if you use her Cleansers.

Foundations — form a base for your make-up. They contain water, oil and wax with added pigments. Oil-free bases often contain synthetic derivatives of oils which are moisturizers. Oil-based bases usually contain no water. All usually contain: zinc stearate, titanium dioxide to provide sun blocks, ultramarine blue, iron oxide, bismuth oxychloride, mica, magnesium aluminum silicate and talc. Before beginning your make-up always cleanse and apply a moisturizer, then apply your base. Choose a make-up base only slightly darker than your own coloring — or even a shade lighter. If it's too dark,

you'll look older and haggard. Patricia Allison's base and
Creative Illusions base are as pure as any I've found. Creative
Illusions offers a matte base, oil-free. They both offer hard to
find pink shades. And both offer a white undercoat which can
be mixed with make-up bases that are too dark for those whose
skin is fair and verges toward pink rather than olive or tan.
Physician's Formula, antiallergenic, can be purchased at drug
stores, and a matte base is available. I love Creative Illusions'
oil-free matte base, no powder necessary. Its oil-free formula
is more holistic than Physician's Formula.

   Face Powder — A good make-up is often spoiled by the
wrong face powder. Powder is used over the base to absorb oil
and create a matte finish. Ingredients: zinc stearate, magnesium aluminum silicate, talc, magnesium silicate. Whatever you use, select from a reliable firm, the better to avoid
unnecessary metals and chemicals. You may avoid powder
altogether if you have a normal skin or if you use a non-oily
matte make-up base. Both Patricia Allison and Creative
Illusions offer a translucent powder. Check Aubrey Organics
at your health store. Aubrey offers several shades of powder.
His label reads: silk powder, aloe vera, henna, allantoin and
natural flower oil. Sounds great! Try it!

   Blushes — Blushes come in powder and cream form.
Usual ingredient is mannitol, which is a form of sugar used
as a thickener. Dextrin, a derivative of cornstarch, is also
used to thicken the powder. The color pigments D & C num-
bers 11 and 17 are frequently used. These colors occasionally
irritate the skin and trigger allergies. Blushes containing
these two pigments should not be used by those with sensitive
skin. If a hay fever type of reaction occurs soon after applying,
do not use again. Seek another brand. Those with acne should
avoid blushes which contain mineral oil, lanolin or Vaseline.

   In health stores you'll find a powdered rouge called *Silken*

Earth, made by Aubrey Organics. The "earth color" is hematite. Hematite is a crystallized mineral which may or may not be good for your skin. I don't know. The rouge contains beet extract for coloring, certainly an improvement over the usual dyes. You'll need a good sable make-up brush for applying. Creative Illusions (address in last chapter) offers both a powder and cake rouge. Or try Patricia Allison's cake rouge. She offers beautiful soft pinks. Apply with a brush. Often a powdered rouge will form blotches of color. I prefer the cake rouge which seems to apply more evenly and naturally. However, at the health stores there are cream rouges which are excellent if you use an oil-based foundation.

Mascara — Available in cream liquid or cake form. Avoid the cream liquid types which promise to lengthen or thicken your lashes, especially if you wear contact lenses. They contain tiny rayon synthetic fibers for thickening or lengthening. These minute fibers could get under the lenses and cause damage to the cornea. This is serious. Some of the mascaras contain acrylates which, if you have sensitive skin, could cause allergic reactions and skin irritations.

All cosmetics increase in bacteria as they age and should never be kept over three months, especially eye mascara. Mascara over three months old contains dangerous bacteria. Naturally occurring bacteria also ages and becomes highly contaminated. If the eyelids contain the least skin eruption or blemish, the mascara bacteria could enter the broken skin, resulting in permanent eye damage, such as corneal ulcer. Some women have actually gone blind from accidentally scratching their eyelids with bacteria-ridden mascara applicators. Buy only one mascara at a time and discard it at the end of three months. Purchase mascara wands often and discard those that are used. Avoid purchasing refillable mascara. It requires using the same wand repeatedly. Do not add saliva to cake mascara. It may contain germs which could be dangerous.

The usual ingredients found in cake or cream type mascara and eye shadow include petrolatum, lanolin, carnauba wax, ceresin, beeswax, stearic acid, propylene glycol, isopropyl myristate, gum tragacanth, water and mythllulose — plus preservatives, perfume and ingredients to lend a shiny, frosted look. All these ingredients have been carefully tested for safety because of the sensitivity of the eye area. Even so, serious damage could result from irritants if mascara is allowed to age, and if such contaminated bacteria enter even the slightest scratch along the eye. Try to find one with the least of these ingredients. Creative Illusions is the best I've found. It even encourages the growth of sparse eyelashes.

For Longer Thicker Eyelashes — Use an eyelash curler before applying mascara. Apply your regular coat of mascara. Allow it to dry for at least three minutes. Apply baby powder or fine face powder to a cotton swab and gently dust over your lashes. Then apply a second coat of mascara over the powder. Repeat the procedure until you have achieved the length and thickness you wish. To avoid clumping mascara, turn your wand up vertically and sweep across your lashes like a windshield wiper. Again, synthetic fibers necessary for lengthening can cause irreparable damage even if you don't wear contact lenses.

Eyeliner — usually contains wax and oil bases, pigments and plasticizing agents, plus low concentrations of preservatives to prevent eye irritation. But because of the small protection, bacteria easily contaminates. So avoid sharing eyeliners. If you are subject to allergies, avoid: carmine, chromium oxide greens, ferric ammonium ferrocyanide and magnesium violet. Do observe if your eyes itch, swell, or are red-rimmed. You could be reacting to the above ingredients. Also acrylic and acrylate copolymer can trigger allergic reactions, even though they are reputed to add luster and thickness to lashes. Read the labels before purchasing. Loreal's may be good for those who react to others. Creative Illusions is excellent. Avoid heavy eyeliners. Make sure the line is fine or that it is smudged. You may want to line the upper lid *under* the lashes, too. Never use black. Choose brown or navy.

Don't wear too much undereye liner — they often make you look like a haggard raccoon. And avoid colors under the eyes. That's only for photographic models. Don't emphasize the upper eye crease with an eyeliner if your eyes are deep set. Choose an eye shadow that contrasts with the color of your eyes.

For Heavier Eyebrows — Apply straight vitamin E oil, available at your health store. Or vitamin E with A and D added. Or add castor oil to the vitamin E-A-D oil. Or lanolin. But apply the lanolin only on the eyebrows. Using on the face could trigger the growth of unwanted hair. Or use Fanie's Herbal Oil with her Fine Line Cream over it. It truly does wonders. Rather than the usual eyebrow pencil, which frequently results in harsh lines, do purchase from your stationery store a thick leaded ebony pencil. One is called the Eberhard Faber Ebony pencil, and   another is Dixon's. Be sure the point is blunt. Small strokes give a natural line to the eyebrow. Blend and lighten with an eyebrow brush. A bad feature of the pencil is that it contains lead — but I know of no eyebrow pencil that doesn't contain lead. Seek for an unleaded pencil at your health store if you wish. Good luck! Don't pluck out too much of your eyebrow. A thin line is dreadful. Strive for a natural line.

Lipstick — usually contain oils, waxes, lanolin, dyes, alcohol, preservatives, often *eosin*, which causes allergic reaction in those with sensitive skin. We've said cosmetics age rapidly, but the oils in lipstick usually don't become rancid for about a year. Discard after that. Both Patricia Allison and Creative Illusions offer hard to find pink shades. You may wish to apply two different shades to achieve the shade which blends with your coloring. First apply a dark shade, blot, then apply a lighter shade over that. For many, it requires the blending of two to achieve the color preferred. You may want to try it. Always apply the dark color first. You may need to apply the top coat several times, blotting in between, to achieve your final color. Do blot and add the top color enough times to lighten the final shade. Nothing is so unattractive as a too-dark lipstick. A softer shade is far more natural and youthful. If you don't wish to use an undercoat of a darker shade, but only want it to last longer without smudging, use a darker lipliner first, dust it with face powder to "set" it, then apply your top coat.

Setting Make-up — After applying make-up, spray your face lightly with chilled bottled water (distilled), or Fanie's Mineral Spray, or a mineral water of your choice. Or pat your face lightly with a pure cotton ball dipped in ice water. This cold water treatment sets the make-up and keeps the face fresh looking for hours. Repeat occasionally all through the day for continued freshness. Spray even over your make-up.

Cosmetic Warnings

1. Women the world over are slowly poisoning their bodies with cosmetics containing toxic levels of metals. Copper, nickel, zinc and lead are found in everything from face powder to eye shadow. These dangerous metals are absorbed through the skin into the bloodstream and the nervous system, resulting in a host of metal-caused syndromes — nervousness, depression, insomnia, mental disturbance, irritability, anemia

and more. Zinc toxification, for instance, affects the entire
endocrine glandular system, especially the pituitary, the master gland. Once the pituitary is imbalanced, it is reasonable
to expect the entire system to react, since the pituitary is the
governing gland of the entire endocrine system. Zinc also can
cause hyperactivity and hyperirritability — in extreme cases,
even schizophrenia. Zinc in cosmetics reacts differently from
the zinc taken as a mineral tablet. Metals should not enter
the system via the skin.

If you wish to avoid toxic reactions from these offending
metals, seek out cosmetics which contain less or none of these
poisons. Since cosmetic manufacturers are now required to
list their ingredients, it may not be too difficult to pinpoint
those to be avoided. If you are not sure concerning your
favorite brand, write to the manufacturer and inquire
whether their brands contain zinc, lead, copper, nickel or
mercury. These are the most toxic metals.

2. When studying the label on a cosmetic, be aware that
ingredients are listed in the order of amount contained. The
major ingredient will be listed first with others following in
lessening quantities. Ingredients must be listed by established uniform names. Specific fragrances need not be listed.
The word "fragrance" is ample. Thus the fragrance in some
cosmetics may contain substances which cause adverse reactions. Try to find all cosmetics and creams without fragrance.

3. Three kinds of cosmetic products are required to carry
appropriate warnings on the labels: — deodorants and
antiperspirants; cosmetics packaged in aerosol containers; and
cosmetics which have not been substantially tested for safety
— such as products with a GRAS listing. Avoid all such cosmetics. GRAS means the ingredients have not yet been
totally approved as safe. GRAS means *generally regarded as
safe.* However, if any of these products result in long-term

damage to your skin or scalp, it's doubtful the manufacturer could be held responsible. Let the buyer beware — and aware.

4. Warnings on aerosol containers alert users to avoid spraying in the eyes and to avoid puncturing. The warning is required on deodorant sprays because adverse reactions, such as itching, rash, burning and blistering often occur — also irritations and even infections. Unusual discharges infrequently cause serious damage. Deodorants and antiperspirants are formidable, either fresh or aged. Antiperspirants are used to check the flow of perspiration, which in itself is a danger to health. Substances employed in such products must affect the body's sweating mechanism. Therefore antiperspirant products usually include the salts of a number of metals. But the most commonly used are the salts of aluminum. Antiperspirants are different from deodorants in that antiperspirants check the flow of perspiration, whereas deodorants prevent body odor. Since body odor usually is the result of bacteria acting on perspiration, most deodorants contain an antibacterial agent strong enough to kill or prevent the growth of bacteria, such as aluminum salts. Occasionally deodorants will contain, in addition, antibacterial agents such as kaolin, zinc stearate and zinc oxide. Most contain alcohol so should not be used immediately after shaving under arms. Antiperspirants are particularly dangerous, since their ingredients also include aluminum chloride, aluminum sulfate, aluminum chlorhydroxide and other aluminum compounds.

To be safe, many now simply apply dampened baking soda under the arm, which certainly acts as an effective deodorant. Also there are now available deodorants containing baking soda. Do choose your deodorant from a health store. They are far less dangerous. Some may be totally free of all dangerous compounds. Or use Fanie's Sweet Birch Cleanser, mentioned earlier, in your daily shower instead of soap. Its daily use will remove all dangerous bacteria which is the cause of odor, so that you don't need to use either a deodorant or antiperspirant.

We all know the current popularity of crystals. So why shouldn't we apply a crystal as a deodorant? As a matter of fact, it is probably the most natural approach available. It's called the *Deodorant Stone* and is probably available at your health store. After a bath or shower, one simply moistens the crystal and applies it underarm or on odorous feet as you would a roll-on deodorant. It prevents odor-causing bacteria from forming. One can't get more natural a methodology than through a crystal. If it is not available at your health store do contact B&K Products. (address in Chapter 10.)

5. As cosmetics age, the controlling preservative in them breaks down and stops working, thus the product becomes contaminated. Applying it to the skin is like applying a live germ culture. Liquid cosmetics are especially dangerous since the germs multiply more rapidly than in dry and solid products, such as powders, lipsticks or eyebrow pencils. Thus you should avoid dipping your fingers into a cream, lotion or powder — or wash the hands before applying. Unwashed hands distribute bacteria in the cream. You may prefer to use sponges or applicators. Store your cosmetics in dry, dark places with lids tightened. Do save the plastic seal which comes atop your cream jar. Replace it after each use to prevent air from circulating inside the jar. Such circulation will breed bacteria.

6. Establish the habit of washing your hands and face thoroughly before touching or applying cosmetics and make sure the cosmetics are applied in clean surroundings. Keep all cosmetic jars or containers tightly closed, avoiding exposure to excessive heat, sunlight or unclean surroundings.

7. Beware of Cosmetic Testers. Don't be tempted to experiment at the store counter with cosmetics which have been used by other people. And don't have a "free demonstration" facial if the make-up artist is using make-up used on previous clients. Dangerous viruses, especially herpes, can be passed along through cosmetics.

Beauty and Make-up Guidelines

Check your make-up with a magnifying mirror near a window. Sunlight picks up many flaws that can be corrected before leaving home.

Use vitamin E ointment on dry skin patches, especially on peeling palms and fingers. Apply it to scars to eventually banish them.

For a quick skin pickup, mix equal portions of fruit juice and milk. Apply to face and throat, leave on ten or fifteen minutes, rinse in tepid water, then apply moisturizer and make-up.

Use equal parts of polarized or mineral water and apple cider vinegar as a skin toner. If sprayed, be sure your eyes are closed.

Don't wear frosted eye shadow. It emphasizes creases. Any frosted substance around the eyes emphasizes crow's feet and fine lines.

Wear lip gloss over your lipstick only in the evening if at all.

Use a lighter moisturizer in summer. Heavy ones just clog pores.

Use lemon juice or witch hazel to abolish pimples. Use witch hazel only on the pimples, not the entire face.

Don't strive for a suntan. It has "gone out of style." Where once a suntan was envied, it now only makes one appear foolish. Instead of impressing, someone with a suntan "falls" in esteem, because one wonders at their level of intelligence. Besides, it isn't really "becoming." It's not natural — and natural is always fashionable.

Don't wear skinny high heels. No one really walks properly in them. You look like you're trying to balance on stilts. Instead of attracting, you only arouse sympathy, because everyone knows you'll spend time at a chiropractor's or osteopath's office to repair your bad back. And you'll increase the problems of childbirth. Also you burn sixty to seventy percent more energy and become tired more easily in high heels. (However, some ladies write to say their leg muscles ache in low heels. To each his own.)

Don't use a man's razor on legs or underarms. Too many nicks. Use a woman's. Or better yet, a good depilatory from your health store.

For foot odor make two cups of tea, using two tea bags. Let them steep for twenty minutes in very hot water. Pour the hot tea into a foot tub containing two quarts of cool water. Soak your feet for twenty to thirty minutes daily for about ten days. No more odorous feet! Repeat once a week or whenever necessary.

Be cautious in wearing pale or colored hose. Colored hose often look gaudy — pale hose look odd unless worn with coordinating colors. Wear traditional natural shades or near black.

Don't wear "stringy" hair! Too "trendy." Some trends look as if the hair was never combed. Or that one washed but forgot to roll it. Or that one deliberately struggled to make hair look tangled and shaggy. It looks like the result of a bad permanent — with eternal frizzled ends. When the trend has passed, I wonder how certain movie stars will feel to see themselves in films looking like a frizzled mop.

Don't wear "dragonlady" nails. They aren't really attractive. And don't wear strange colored polish — such as white or black. Looks gruesome. Don't wear false nails unless they're the thin kind. The thick ones make hands look like claws.

Don't wear hi-cut panties or girdles under polyester pants. They make a line and indentation, spoiling a clean-line effect. Choose pantyhose with spandex or a long-legged panty or girdle.

Don't wear huge shoulder pads, no matter what the movie stars are wearing in movies. It's a passing fad. If you must wear them, be sure they are moderate and accentuate your shoulder width, not increase it beyond natural lines.

Don't wear the belt that came with the dress, unless it's highly attractive. Exchange for one that's more attractive. A beautiful belt can change your dress from drab or "dowdy" to striking appeal.

Don't wear gaudy necklaces or earrings. Even the most expensive make you look pretentious, as if you're trying to compensate or showoff for lack of innate qualities.

Don't pierce your ears! It's downright dangerous. The hole pierces right through a most important acupuncture point. Keeping that point constantly aggravated or stimulated by metal is or can be deadly. If you suffer from some unknown health problem, it could be caused by your bejeweled pierced ears.

Chapter Six

Hair —
Our Crowning Glory

Human hair cells grow seven times faster than other cells. Thus it would seem that nutritional deficiencies seriously affect the growth of hair and its appearance more rapidly than any other part of the anatomy, unless it would be the fingernails. Hair reflects internal as well as external well-being. Vitamins, minerals, enzymes, protein and the proper carbohydrates are vital to the manufacture of hair cells and their life span.

The B vitamins are especially essential. Niacin is vital to circulation. Biotin is recognized as an absolute essential to hair growth, maintenance, and even restoration. Folic acid is essential to the building process of RNA. B12 is vital to normal cell growth. You can obtain a vitamin B extract containing the total vitamin complex from Fanie, a few drops daily under the tongue. Or take yeast tablets. Minerals are equally essential — especially iron, copper, zinc and silica. Copper is important in maintaining hair color and zinc is vital to the formation of hair cells. (Not the same as zinc used in cosmetics.) Silica is probably the most important mineral for healthy hair and nails. Deficiency, therefore, in vitamins, minerals and enzymes can be disastrous, together with the deleterious effect of permanents, blow dryers, dyes, shampoos and even the abuses of sunlight.

Since hair is a vital part of the whole person it cannot be treated as a separate item. Hair is an integrated unit as much a part of your total being as your nails, skin or eyes. Falling hair is usually the result of concentrations of toxic wastes in the body, concentrations of male hormones on the scalp, drugs and chemicals in medications, and pollutions in the diet. It is well, of course, to be aware of external hair preparations and efforts to restore hair to its ultimate glory, but it is also well to be aware that hair, a gauge of the body's well-being, may be maintained through a proper purification program which will affect not only the hair but the entire being — a purification program involving ridding the body of its toxic wastes — which may mean a partial fast — then entering a regimen of healthy eating, thinking and exercising. Prevention is seldom popular with the masses, but one would do well to think about beautiful hair long before it seems necessary. In other words, it is not wise to wait until hair loss is obvious before beginning a program of restoration and purification for the whole person, thereby never needing to worry about hair loss, or lack of beauty.

The Anatomy of Hair

To understand the cause of hair loss and to prevent it, it is well to know how the hair itself is formed, how it is nourished, and the conditions favorable or unfavorable to its growth. Having learned this, the methods by which its loss can be arrested and vitality regained may be more readily comprehended and successfully practiced.

The hair is a tube composed of the same elements as the nails or the bones. The secretions by which all three are formed are the same and they do not appear to decrease as age advances. Therefore, the major cause of hair loss would seem to be, and usually is, local. Hair is composed of three layers. First, the outer layer of transparent cells which lie one upon the other like shingles on a roof. This layer, called the follicle, protects the second layer, called the cortex or shaft. The shaft is filled with minuscule vortices through which natural oils give the hair its sheen. It is through these vortices that the natural coloring matter is drawn up through the scalp. The coloring matter is then reflected through the outer follicle. The third layer is called the canal or medulla, forming the strong core of the hair.

Technically, hairs do not have roots, but at the end of the hair embedded in the scalp is found a miniature bulb often called the hair root. This bulb encloses the papilla, the opening through which the hair receives its nourishment from the bloodstream. For lack of a better word, "root" will be used in these writings. Often when a hair is pulled from the scalp, the bulb or root is visible. But the papilla always remains inside the scalp. As long as the papilla can receive nourishment from the bloodstream the hair continues to live, to fall out, and to be replaced by another living hair. Thus, hair consists ultimately of a root and a shaft, enclosed in a narrow cavity known as the follicle. Surrounding the hair follicle, also, are the sebaceous and sweat glands. The sebaceous secretes oils while the sweat glands produce, obviously, perspiration. When the oil is mixed with grime and debris which blocks the glands and arteries of the scalp, it is called sebum. Exces-

sive cholesterol helps to create the sebum, which plugs the
arteries and prevents blood from reaching the hair roots,
much as hardened oil blocks the arteries throughout the
body. The hair follicle is also surrounded by nerves through
which flow a nerve force, recognized as prana, or life force.

Thus, we are made aware that hair loss is often
attributed to blood loss in the scalp because of hardened
sebum. Without the flow of nutritional blood, the hair
cannot grow. The usual growth rate is about 3/4 of an inch
a month. First, feed the bloodstream the proper nutrients,
then feed your hair follicles with a free flowing bloodstream. Again, the condition of the hair and nails is one
of the first reflections of ill health, indicating that something is inadequate in the metabolism. Nails become dry,
brittle and perpetually break. The hair also becomes dry,
brittle and lifeless, and ultimately falls out, not to be
replaced. One of the first steps to regain hair or prevent
the loss is to remove that which is obstructing the flow of
blood in the scalp. It might be well to think of adding
flaxseed oil to your diet — which could loosen and destroy
the sebum in the scalp which is causing the obstruction —
just as flaxseed or cod liver oil removes hardened deposits
in the arteries to prevent heart attacks.

The Cause of Hair Loss

The theory that baldness is caused by heredity is incor-
rect. Heredity simply cannot be blamed. If heredity were
the cause, then why would not all the children of a given
set of parents become bald? If one of the sons of these parents becomes bald, then why not *all* the sons? It could be
said that one brother inherited genes from the father and
the other from the mother. But what of the parents with

full heads of hair who have bald sons? If one son is bald, then why not all the sisters? Yet this doesn't happen. Brothers and sisters often do not reflect the same hair problems. Seldom do the sisters become bald. Thus, heredity is not acceptable. A list of causes is offered:

1. the diet
2. vitamin deficiency and defective circulation
3. uncleanliness of the scalp
4. failure to remove dead hairs which impedes the growth of new ones
5. excessive testosterone, a male hormone
6. excessive estrogen, a female hormone
7. birth control pills
8. accumulated cholesterol in the scalp which enter the sebaceous glands and arteries, hardening as sebum to block the flow of nutrients to the hair and scalp
9. thyroid gland deficiency
10. tight or heavy hats
11. tight collars and neckties which restrict the flow of blood to the scalp
12. anemia, a blood condition (iron deficiency)
13. excessive vitamin A
14. exposure to certain chemicals
15. certain feminine hair fashions
16. dissipation
17. sexual excess
18. weakness of the muscles which are attached to the hair
19. microbes or germ diseases in the scalp
20. deficiency of calcium, zinc, vitamin B and silica

Any one or all of these may produce baldness. If you remove the cause or causes, and follow the simple direc-

tions contained in this writing, there is every possibility
of avoiding baldness or restoring at least a partial head of
hair. Since practicing the system of physical exercises
offered by Sanford Bennett will surely result in improvement in the general condition of the entire body, they will
also contribute toward a proportionate improvement in the
health of the hair. (See *The Book of Beginning Again*.)
Let's consider each of the causes just listed.

The Diet

Foods to especially avoid are: refined white salt, refined
white sugar, white flour, and excessive animal fats. Also
avoid excessive alcohol and tobacco. *Refined white salt* crys-
tallizes in the blood capillaries in the scalp, closing off and
restricting the blood supply. Substitute a total mineral
salt or vegetable salt (Real Salt or Dews Salt) and begin
the corrective measures described later, which will break
up the blockages of accumulated salt crystals. *Refined
white sugar*, white flour and alcohol destroy the B vitamins.
Loss of the B vitamins results in baldness. Substitute
Dews sugar or date sugar. (See last chapter.) *Tobacco* con-
stricts blood capillaries, reducing the circulation especially
across the scalp. *Excessive intake of animal fats* affects the
normal functioning of the sebaceous glands in the scalp.

Since foreign chemicals in the body cause baldness, it
is well to eliminate *all processed foods* containing preservatives, additives and dyes, and turn to a more natural
diet. Foods to avoid include fried foods, hydrogenated oils,
hot dogs, corned beef, lunch meats, bacon, ham, cola drinks,
soft drinks, tea, coffee, chocolate, some cereals, frozen TV
dinners, desserts (pies, cakes), and foods containing
monosodium glutamate, sulfur dioxide and benzoate of

soda. Remember, your hair is affected by the food you eat.

Vitamin-Mineral Deficiency and Defective Circulation

Since hair is composed entirely of protein, it requires protein to grow. Essential amino acids compose the natural formula of proteins. The principal amino acid required for the growth of hair is *cystine*. This amino acid must enter the body through food. Your blood supply cannot deliver the required nutrients to your hair unless the nutrients are supplied by your diet. Thus it is often wise to supplement the diet with a natural vitamin-mineral-enzyme tablet, and amino acid capsules. Again, especially needed are the B vitamins — biotin, pantothenic acid, para-aminobenzoic acid, inositol, folic acid and nicotinic acid. A teaspoon of pure inositol each day has aided in restoring hair.

Vitamin B deficiency creates an alteration in the content of lactose and lactic acid in the blood flow to the brain cells, so necessary for the brain to build food into cells and mental energy. Vitamin B deficiency creates hardening of the arteries of the brain which means a decreased flow of oxygenated blood to the brain cells and hair follicles. Nicotinic acid, a B vitamin, also has a dilating effect on blood vessels and could very well stimulate hair growth by increasing the blood supply through dilated blood vessels in the scalp (nicotinic acid, usually called *niacin*, has nothing whatever to do with nicotine, a deadly poison found in tobacco).

Dry brittle hair is often an indication of vitamin A deficiency, but do not take Vitamin A to excess. It stimulates the action of the sebaceous glands and overstimulation could cause hair loss. Take vitamin A in the form of Beta Carotene. Vitamin E dilates blood vessels and increases the blood flow to the skin surface. It also oxygenates the blood and stimulates the circulation. Vitamin F, found in cold pressed unrefined vegetable oils, stimulates the flow of sebum from the sebaceous glands, aiding in the restoration of hair growth. Flaxseed oil and cod liver oil are also aids in dissolving the hardened sebum in the arteries of the head.

Essential minerals — such as silica, zinc, iodine, calcium, and iron to avoid anemia — can be supplied with kelp tablets. Kelp also contains magnesium, phosphorus, potassium, and copper. But the nutrients in the diet, or a hair vitamin-mineral tablet, will not result in hair growth unless the small blood capillaries in your scalp are supplied with the flow of blood. The exercises later described will do much to aid that achievement.

Cleanliness

Perspiration has a very injurious effect upon the hair. Athletes are especially subject to this threat. They usually terminate athletic activities with perspiration exuding from every pore, the hair being equally saturated. The poisonous dead matter should be shampooed out before it dries upon the scalp and hair. Men are far more prone to scalp perspiration than women.

Brushing and Grooming

When the hair is falling out, many refrain from properly brushing for fear of causing more hair loss. This is a serious mistake. Dead hair roots, like any other decaying matter, are injurious to the healthy roots near them and, if allowed to remain, increase the trouble. They should be removed from their healthy neighbors. Dead and decaying matter is a menace to the life of a hair just as, upon a larger scale, dead matter and unsanitary conditions are a menace to the life of a human being.

In addition to injurious effects of the dead roots, they impede the growth of new hairs which would spring up in place of the dead ones, but which cannot do so while dead roots remain. Remove the dead hairs as soon as possible and other healthy hairs will replace them, springing from the same follicles or root sheath. Daily brushing is a must. Each time combing and brushing is performed, there is a natural loss of hair. This is perfectly normal, and should not be of concern. Details of hair brushing will be given later.

Alas, Which Shampoo?

The scalp, similar to any other part of the body, is filled with thousands of little pores which are constantly eliminating refuse matter. In addition, the sebaceous glands throw off sebum oil which adheres to the scalp. This debris must be removed or the pores will be clogged, a condition which is very injurious. The scalp should be thoroughly cleaned at least once a week, preferably twice, and for some perhaps even daily.

How often one washes the hair is a personal matter. Some insist their hair thrives on daily shampoos. Others find the daily washing results in a dry, lifeless condition, the frequency of the shampoo removing all the natural oil. Some find twice a week adequate, while others retain the once-a-week routine. If one indulges in daily scalp massage and brushing, once or twice a week shampooing may be sufficient. This enables the natural hair oil to saturate the hair with a natural sheen. Each individual must decide how his or her hair responds to the frequency of shampoos.

Thousands lose their hair through neglecting cleanliness and it is far better to shampoo daily than to neglect cleanliness. Always brush the hair and massage the scalp just before shampooing. The brushing will remove dead hairs and much of the greasy impurities. Try applying warm jojoba or castor oil to the scalp before shampooing. Then wrap the hair in a warm damp towel and allow it to steam for at least 10 minutes. Remove the towel and allow the oil to remain another 20 minutes. Or wrap the head in a dry towel and leave on overnight. Or cover the head with a plastic shower cap to insure heat. Three soapings of shampoo may be required to remove all the grease and grime loosened by the oil treatment.

Most shampoos now available are to be avoided. They are strong in alkali and their oil content may be rancid. They may also contain synthetic perfume, synthetic oils, and sulfur mixes. Many shampoos list the following ingredients: FD and C Yellow No. 5, FD and C Yellow No. 6, FD and C Red No. 40, FD and C Blue No. 2, Red Dye No. 2, Blue Dye No. 1. Here is an analysis of these color additives. Read it and turn gray: FD and C Yellow No. 5: a coal tar derivative which, in itself, is enough to cause you to toss away your shampoo. It has the approval of the FDA even though it causes allergic reactions such as wheezing, asthmatic symptoms, and hives. FD and C Yellow No. 6: a coal tar product, causing all allergic reactions recognized as sensitive to coal tar. Approved by the FDA. FD and C Blue No. 2: causes allergic reactions so serious it is not permitted in hypoallergenic cosmetics. Red Dye No. 2 and Blue Dye No. 1 produced tumors in test animals. They can cause serious allergic reactions.

When possible, avoid all color additives, chiefly those that are coal tar derivatives. Especially avoid using them around the eyes. All coal tar colors are suspect because, in tests, all have been shown to cause cancer when injected into the skin of mice. Also, many people have violent allergic reactions. Six permanently listed coal tar colors are, at the moment, approved and considered safe. Others are on the provisional or GRAS list — which means the FDA is awaiting further results of toxicity or safety.

Many modern shampoos contain synthetic detergents. Before synthetic detergents became popular, plain soap was used as a shampoo. But soap is usually alkaline and will not perform well in hard water. Hard water contains a relatively high amount of calcium which reacts with the alkaline soap to form deposits of a gummy residue called "soap scum." (The familiar ring in the bathtub is formed by deposits of calcium, soap and dirt.) Soap combining with hard water can form undissolved scum on the hair during shampooing. It not only dulls the luster but makes it difficult to comb. Thus synthetic detergents have become popular in shampoos because of their ability to mix with hard water, and that they do not form soap scum.

However, synthetic detergents in shampoos are often dangerous. They are classified as anionic, cationic, nonionic or amphoteric, depending on the action of ions in water. Shampoos sold for adults usually contain synthetic detergents of the anionic type. Shampoos for babies and children contain the amphoteric type, often mixed with anionic type. Synthetic detergents of the cationic type are extremely dangerous in shampoos and were once known to cause severe eye damage and often permanent injury. Even now it is not unusual to experience allergenic skin reactions, such as watery eyes or itching scalp. Read the label carefully on your shampoo. If uncertain, contact the manufacturer to inquire the type of synthetic detergent used in the product. Soap is still being used for shampooing, the scum being removable by rinsing with apple cider vinegar or lemon juice as described later. It may still be advisable to use these rinses even when a synthetic detergent shampoo is used.

What is one to do? The synthetic detergent is used to thoroughly remove the soap scum, yet the stronger the detergent the more apt it is to irritate the scalp and damage the natural oil flow. You may prefer to choose a baby shampoo which is usually formulated from amphoteric synthetic detergents which are comparatively non-irritating and stingless. But such shampoos are not expected to remove deposits of hair sprays or other prior hair products. Most baby shampoos result in minimum irritation.

Or search the shelves at your health store for pure herbal solutions — such as *Ma Evans Herbal Hair Lotion*. (See last chapter for sources if unavailable at your local health store.)

Or you may want to choose Fanie's Oak Bark Shampoo and her once a week Oak Bark Hair Treatment. They are totally natural, containing *no* detergents. They are the finest I've ever found, and I'd never think of using anything else. The weekly Hair Treatment certainly worked wonders on my thinning hair. The oak bark, a natural DMSO, penetrates where the sebum is blocking the cells and glands, preventing the flow of blood. It dissolves the encrusted sebum. Once the sebum is destroyed, the blood flow brings nutrients to the hair and new hair grows. My once thinning hair is now fairly full again.

The effects of white oak bark were well known to the ancients. Different parts of the tree were used, but it is the bark which is now used in natural and holistic medicines. Compounded with PCMX, as are Fanie's products, they are without a doubt the most effective known skin and scalp antiseptic type cleanser, plus the white oak pulp containment of DMSO wetting solvents and penetrating activities. Added to this are herbs proven to be effective in baldness, thinning hair, scalp exfoliation and in some diseases of the scalp. These include rosemary, basil, parsley, nettle, sage, goldenseal, alfalfa, comfrey, dandelion, kelp, cayenne, and garlic. Each herb, containing natural portions of vitamin A, B complex, vitamin C, niacin, and minerals in their natural state, are formulated with the white oak bark solution.

Rosemary has been used over 3,000 years to combat baldness, thinning hair and scalp problems. Basil contains methylchavical, eucalyptol, linalook, estragal — all used effectively for thinning hair for over 2,000 years. Parsley contains calcium, magnesium, phosphorous, potassium, sodium, together with vitamin A (22 times more than carrots), vitamin C (three times more than lemons), iron (five times more than spinach), vitamin B complex, folic acid, niacin, pantothenic acid. All these marvelous God-made solutions are carried deep into the cells through the DMSO action of the pulp of white oak bark.

Conditioners often include synthetic eggs, proteinaceous substances, protein derivatives, glycerin or propylene glycol and ethyl alcohol. When using the Fanie products no conditioner is necessary, which is another reason for their effectiveness. If interested, see the last chapter for where to order.

If you prefer to use the usual drug store shampoo, brunettes should follow the shampoo with a rinse of apple cider vinegar. The solution should be two tablespoons of vinegar to a pint of warm water. This vinegar rinse removes the last particles of soap that may be left on the hair. Be sure to rinse out all the vinegar. Blondes should use a lemon rinse which lightens the color, whereas vinegar rinses darken the hair for the brunette. The lemon formula is the juice of one lemon in a pint of warm water.

Regardless your choice of shampoo, each washing should be followed with a hot water rinse, then a cold water rinse — a strong stimulant to blood circulation. The application of hot water draws the blood toward the surface, the cold drives it back and inward. The surging of the blood toward the surface and back not only stimulates circulation but oxygenizes the scalp cells and even the hair itself. Alternate the water half a dozen times, allowing each application to thoroughly permeate the entire surface of the head before changing the water temperature. Have the temperature of the heated water as hot as you can bear it, and the other as cold as possible. If life still remains in the roots of the hair a healthy growth will usually result. The tonic effect of this process is far more efficacious than any medicinal hair invigorator yet invented. End with the cold temperature.

Always blot-dry the hair thoroughly with a towel. Then, if possible, continue to dry outside in the fresh air and sunshine. When almost dry, a few drops of coconut or sweet almond oil will produce an attractive and healthy gloss.

For best results roll the hair when almost dry, then spray with a mist spray bottle. Allow hair to dry naturally — for instance, overnight. There are "spongy" rollers available for overnight sleeping. Never use artificial heat unless absolutely necessary. Use mild heat, never hot, as hot ruins not only hair, but facial skin. It is best never to blow dry your hair — the steady stream of artificial heat is devastating to hair health. If you must blow dry, be sure your hand-held dryer has a mica lining and not asbestos. Mica, though not altogether safe, is better than asbestos, particles of which, inhaled regularly, could cause lung cancer.

Sebum and Hair Loss

A major cause of hair loss is an excessive buildup of sebum on the scalp. When natural oil discharged by the sebaceous gland is filled with cholesterol and other debris, it becomes sebum. With a buildup of sebum, baldness usually results. Sebum is a waxy oil which dries and hardens in the arteries and follicles of the scalp. It lies in several microscopic layers. Sebum, once thought to be a natural lubricant of the scalp, actually is a form of body waste, much like the oil that seeps on the facial areas of a person with acne. Also it is highly acid which, drying on the scalp, results in dandruff.

When excessive sebum is discharged the follicles become clogged. Hardening in the follicles, much as cholesterol hardens in the arteries, gradually destroys the cuticle which holds the hair in place. Eventually, it causes the hair to fall out, not to be replaced. Its continuing excessive flow becomes a bacteria that finally destroys hair roots. Once this occurs the follicle can no longer give birth to hair. Dandruff is the first symptom of a sebum related problem, followed by excessively oily hair, itchiness of the scalp, greasy forehead and the common ring around the collar. Often itchy bumps may appear on the scalp. Although all baldness is not sebum related, it is to blame in the majority of cases.

Testosterone, a Male Hormone

A male hormone called testosterone causes hair loss under certain conditions. Testosterone hormones are quite natural in both the male and female, but flows more abundantly in the male. It becomes a problem in hair loss when it accumulates in the tissues of the scalp and the hair follicles — and the substance responsible for the excessive accumulation is cholesterol. Cholesterol is believed to transform into the hormone testosterone through a process called biosynthesis in the dermal tissues of the scalp. For some unknown reason, the glands of the scalp attract and store cholesterol. When cholesterol accumulates in the tissues it attracts an overabundance of testosterone which, in turn, causes a blockage of the flow of pranic life force and fresh oxygenated blood to the scalp. The flow of excessive testosterone stimulates the sebaceous glands, resulting in overabundance of sebum, the scalp skin oil. Sebum becomes encrusted in the hair follicles, preventing the growth of new hair. In experiments with rabbits and mice, when sebum is painted on the skin, hair is lost in 10 days. The exercises offered later break up scalp cholesterol and loosen the subcutaneous tissue surrounding hair follicles, resulting in increased blood circulation in the capillary system of the scalp. Taking flaxseed oil daily could also be extremely beneficial in dissolving the hardened sebum. See *The You Book* for full information concerning the diet and a buildup of cholesterol — homogenized milk, for example. A change in diet could change the entire "balding" pattern.

Estrogen and Birth Control Pills

Women should be equally aware of the possibility of hair loss via birth control pills, which flood the body with excessive estrogen, a female hormone — just as an overabundance of the male hormone, testosterone, causes loss of hair. Other hazards connected with The Pill are: thick curly hair straightens and becomes limp; dandruff begins and becomes excessive; the skin around the vagina becomes irritated; the complexion changes — pimples and blemishes persist where once the skin was clear. Not so obvious effects are vitamins A and C deficiencies, exposing one to infections and allergies. Also a deficiency in B vitamins results, especially B1, B6, B12 and folic acid.

The Pill equally robs the body of important minerals, especially iron and zinc. Continued usage could lead to diabetes, gall bladder problems, kidney failure, edema, liver congestion, high blood pressure, varicose veins, thrombophlebitis (blood clots), heart attacks and cancer of the cervix and breast. In Chapter 4 I have suggested an alternative to The Pill.

Hair loss also often occurs through insufficient estrogen after menopause. Estrogen deficiencies can often be corrected with herbal capsules which can be an excellent substitute for estrogen therapy. Take it cautiously. A resulting headache could indicate you are receiving an overabundance of estrogen. Consider also a product called G+, herbal capsules containing cedar berries and ginseng, available from Dynapro International, Inc., (address in last chapter). It is offered to women who, following a hysterectomy, cannot or do not wish to continue estrogen therapy. The allopathic estrogen therapy usually focuses on *Premarin*, the source of which is said to be a pregnant mare.

If Premarin is your choice do try the weakest, which are the green tablets. Next in strength are the brown tablets. The strongest are purple, which could cause excessive estrogen in the body.

Youth, the Thyroid Gland, and Gray Hair

The secret of a long life may lie principally in preserving a healthy condition of the thyroid gland. The thyroid is the small gland situated at the lower part of the throat. As every organ of the body has its special duty to perform, it may be that, aside from being a factor in our general health, one of the functions of the thyroid is to secrete the coloring pigment of the hair. Read what Sanford Bennett had to say about the thyroid and gray hair:

"After three months practice in stimulating this gland by massage, combined with the throat muscle exercises, I found that my hair became much darker in patches and strips. After discontinuing the exercises for two weeks, the color disappeared. I then commenced again and, in about a week more, nearly all of the same results were obtained. Whether degeneration of the thyroid is the principal cause of gray hair, or whether the original color can be permanently regained by stimulating it to activity by massage, in connection with exercises of the surrounding muscles, is an interesting experiment. There is one thing certain, the coloring of the hair must be secreted by some gland and it is just possible it is the thyroid."

Unless an overactive thyroid is indicated, do take kelp capsules to supply iodine and important minerals and amino acids.

An oriental method of stimulating the thyroid not only may return the color of the hair and prevent baldness, but will add to the regeneration of the entire body. Master Sehan Kim, the Oriental acupuncturist who taught it to me, called it the "Youthifier." He is mentioned at length in *The Book of Beginning Again*. Master Kim claimed this technique kept the body young. Place the thumb and fore-finger of either hand upon the throat, one on each side of the "Adam's apple." Locate the pulse point on each side, moving the fingers until the pulse point is found. Apply pressure first with the thumb on one pulse point and hold to the pulse count of seven. Release and press with the forefinger or first two fingers on the pulse point on the other side of the throat. Again hold to the pulse count of seven. Alternate back and forth between pressure upon the pulse with the thumb and pressure with the fingers from 10 to 15 minutes. Always hold to the pulse count of seven. Repeated daily, this regulates the action of the thyroid and releases important hormones into the bloodstream. The stimulation of the thyroid may well restore the hair's nat-ural coloring.

Another proven method of restoring or maintaining natural color: take 200 mg. of PABA after each meal. The coloring matter of the hair is generated in the hair bulb and from there forced up the tubular hair shaft. The char-acter of the scalp secretions determine the color of the hair. The chemical combinations which produce that color are not known. But as years go by, there is evidently a chem-ical change in the secretions which cause a loss of the col-oring matter. Loss of color can result from a lack of min-erals in the diet. Copper is particularly essential to main-tain natural hair color. Natural color has also been restored through vitamin therapy — pantothenic acid, para-aminobenzoic acid (PABA), folic acid, nucleic acid and vitamin E. On the other hand, *sulfa drugs* have been known to bring about instantaneous gray hair (not natural sulfur). It is known to destroy the body's store of pantothenic acid, a deficiency of which causes the loss of hair color. *Gerovital* (GH3) is renowned for restoring the loss of hair and the color. You'll find full information later in this chapter. See the last chapter for where to order.

Conventional Male Fashions — Shirts, Ties, Hats

Another cause of hair loss in the male could possibly be wearing tight-collared shirts. Men — victims of a fashion-minded world which requires wearing shirts which bind the neck, and neckties which add to that binding — may find themselves not only experiencing bizarre episodes of dizziness, but possibly the restriction of blood supply to the brain which may cause the loss of hair. Tight ties can also affect the eyesight. Tests with tight ties at the College of Human Ecology at Cornell University found that such neckwear causes a loss of visual perception, harming the performance of computer operators, airplane pilots and others who require good visual discrimination. Experiment with larger shirt sizes and resist tightening the necktie beyond adequacy. Defy convention as often as possible in favor of "casual" garments. Toss away your hats. They no longer seem a necessary part of the male wardrobe, except in colder climates or as a covering when exposed to sun rays.

Hair Dyes and Cosmetics

The oily secretion of the sebaceous glands makes a valiant effort to protect the scalp against the invasion of foreign substances. But many of the substances used in hair cosmetics are capable of destroying the defensive barriers and seep into the living cells beneath the scalp tissues. Among the worst offenders are the metals found in shampoos, hair rinses, dyes, tints, conditioners, wave lotions, bleaches, lacquers, and chemical hair sprays. In almost all these solutions are found nickel, aluminum, mercury, lead, tin and silver, all extremely dangerous not only for the scalp, but for the very life force itself if enough accumulates. Hair dyes also contain metallic salts such as copper, lead, and iron, in addition to aniline dyes, plus aminophenols and paradiamino-benzenes. These dyes and chemicals accumulate as a poisonous substance in the blood, kidneys and liver, resulting in aniline poisoning and, often, in mental problems, loss of memory, confusion, loss of emotional control. It is strongly suggested that one avoid hair dyes completely. Tests also strongly indicate that several hair dye chemicals may cause cancer. They have been shown to damage genes, resulting in cancer or birth defects in offspring.

In some hair dyes vegetable coloring is used, such as henna, indigo, camomile, sage, nutgall. These vegetable colors are far safer than the hair dyes, tints, and rinses that contain coal tar or aniline colors, which not only frequently cause allergic reactions but, entering the bloodstream through osmosis, carry a threat of systemic poisoning, especially if the dyes are combined with peroxide compounds. Inquire of your beauty operator if your hair dye contains coal tar dyes. Most coal tar products have proven to be cancer-causing.

If you once prove allergic to paraphenylene-diamine-type dye, never again submit to its usage. This chemical dye is used in making coal tar colors, the final color being produced by oxidizing this chemical. Any coal tar hair products are also hazardous if used around the eyes. Numerous eye injuries have resulted from their use in eye shadow and mascara. Some of these dangerous substances are: resorcinol, arsenic, tar, sulfonamides, quinine, glycerin, resin of maleic, anhydride, chlorine or oxalic acid. . . any one of which may cause severe allergic reaction or dermatitis. Before submitting to any kind of hair dye it is well to run an allergy test by applying a small portion to a patch of freshly washed and dried skin, usually on the inner side of an elbow. The substance should dry on the skin and be left undisturbed for 24 hours. If itching, burning, rash, inflammation or irritation results, the product should never be used.

Of course, the patch test is satisfactory only for those who are at that moment sensitive and allergic to the substance. It is of little help to those who will become sensitive and allergic as the dye is persistently used. If you frequently dye your hair be alert to notice any kind of inflammation on the skin, whether on the scalp or not — any irritation, rash, eruptions of any kind. Should you become aware of such a problem immediately consult a dermatologist and ask for an allergy test of your particular hair dye. In the event you find yourself suddenly allergic to the dye already on your hair, immediately begin daily shampoos to remove as much of the dye as possible. Consider thoroughly rinsing the hair with hydrogen peroxide solution to oxidize any residual dye, removing the peroxide, of course, with a shampoo. If your dermatologist advises against this, it may even be necessary to crop the hair closely to the scalp, ridding yourself of as much of the dangerous substance as is possible.

Hair dye frequently contains lead and can very well result in lead poisoning, surfacing as any number of unexplainable complaints such as headaches, arthritis and even mental problems. So if you are suffering from any of these related symptoms, or even a loss of memory and confusion, better see a doctor or dermatologist about a hair analysis. If an abundance of lead is found, you have possibly located the cause of your problem.

It is not uncommon to suddenly discover one's hair is turning green. Have you been swimming in a swimming pool recently? Green hair indicates excess copper in the water of the pool that saturates and reacts upon the hair. Shampoo daily until hair color returns to normalcy and immediately remove the excess copper from the pool water.

Hair Sprays and Treatments

In 1987, 47,000 cases of injuries caused by cosmetics were reported by hospital emergency staffs to the Consumer Product Safety Commission. Many hair sprays and treatments cause asthma, dizziness and loss of memory, and make it easy for hair to ignite. Other complaints include respiratory problems, skin diseases, headaches and nausea. And miscarriages should be included. Even ingredients the FDA has found to be toxic or carcinogenic (cancer-causing) — such as methyl chloride used in hair spray and methacrylate used to create sculptured fingernails — are still in use both in salon products and in products sold to consumers.

Feminine Hair Fashions

Loss of hair among women might also be traced to hair fashions. Tight braids and "pony tails" can create a strain upon the hair shaft, apparently causing the hair follicles to regress and become inflamed, resulting in baldness.

Even worse, standard practice is to "tease" the hair so that the "hairdo" lasts from week to week, resulting in very little combing, no brushing and no scalp stimulation. On the day of the beauty salon appointment, the hair is shampooed and often dried with a hot air blower . . . a sure avenue towards loss of hair later. To add to the risk, the cloud of chemical hair spray, in which the face and head is enveloped, not only affects the lungs but damages the hair and skin as, week after week, the hair undergoes its torturous routine. The hair spray contains synthetic resins which accumulate in the lungs, lymph nodes, liver, spleen and other organs, also affecting the eyes, skin and, possibly, the hearing. Entering the ear canal, inflammation of the canal and possible deafness could be the result.

The cold wave permanent has also contributed to hair loss among females. The chemical required to produce the curl, usually thioglycate, is extremely detrimental to hair, the hair shaft, hair follicles and scalp. More than one unfortunate woman has experienced temporary baldness due to reaction to permanent wave solutions. The neutralizing solution, containing potassium bromide, a highly toxic substance, has more than once accidentally entered the ear, perforating the ear drum and resulting in loss of hearing.

A happy note is that cosmetic laboratories are constantly seeking for less toxic approaches for our beautification. Among the promising products is *Panthenol*, a pro-vitamin that the body transforms into pantothenic acid, a substance remarkably effective both for hair beauty and skin. *Biotin* products are fast becoming recognized as an important adjunct, especially for hair beauty. Biotin is a B vitamin.

Much is being promised through the use of *kerotin pro-*

tein, too, for hair beauty. Kerotin is the structural protein of which our hair and nails are actually composed. Shampoos containing kerotin protein offer the benefit of 20 amino acids, whereas collagen protein, the basis of most cosmetics, provides only one. An herb called *henna*, a natural hair dye, has been on the cosmetic scene since the days of ancient Egypt, when Egyptian royalty and lay people alike used it generously for hair health and coloring. It is also possible to apply a henna shampoo for hair growth and beauty without changing one's natural coloring. Becoming available, too, are permanent wave solutions free of thioglycolic acid or its salts. Since an overabundance of these metals are deadly, it is happy news to know there are being developed products free of their toxins.

Dandruff

Every head of hair has dandruff since dandruff is the sloughing off of particles of the scarf skin — dead and discarded cells of the scalp. This sloughing off is as normal as is the peeling and renewing of the outer layer of body skin. Nature herself is constantly removing dead cells all over the body, including the scalp. Hence it is perfectly normal for dandruff, or dead cells, to fall. It is more noticeable in the scalp because it frequently accumulates more obviously there than elsewhere because of the flow of oil emitted by the sebaceous glands which, adhering to the scalp and absorbing dirt, dust and smog pollution from the atmosphere, becomes sebum.

That which is usually described as dandruff is *seborrhea*, which is excessive discharges of sebum. Sebum flows naturally along the scalp and into the hair. But when the discharge becomes too copious it sheds as dead cells, flaking

off as seborrhea. Dandruff, then, is the normal shedding
of the outer dead cells of the scalp and everyone experiences
it. In most people it is not obvious, since the exfoliation
is not normally abundant. The particles of scarf skin are
so tenuous as to be unobservable, exfoliating in extremely
fine essences. Seborrhea, on the other hand, is more obvious
since it is an excess of oil sebum combined with the
sloughed off dead layers of scarf skin — the dust, germs
and smog pollution. Seborrhea Oleosa, appearing as dandruff, indicates a malfunction of the sebaceous glands,
emitting an overabundance of the sebum oil — or the opposite, a scaly sloughing off indicating a need for *more* oil.
Brushing and stimulating the scalp through the exercise
given later will usually stabilize the flow of the sebum oil,
overcoming the problem of seborrhea.

Be aware, however, that seborrhea may indicate a vitamin B deficiency, especially B6, biotin and riboflavin. But
do take a vitamin B complex tablet, yeast tablet, or tincture
containing *all* the B family. To take a B vitamin separate
from the entire complex of the B family only means the body
responds with evidence of imbalance. Do also eliminate
white sugar and all foods containing it. They destroy vitamin B in the system, thus often causing seborrhea. Here
is a "home" remedy for dandruff which is far better than
anything bought over-the-counter. Mix equal parts of apple
cider vinegar with water — mineral water or rain water if
possible. Separate the hair in sections and apply the lotion
with pure cotton balls. Follow with your favorite shampoo.
You should soon see a healthier head of hair and gradually
diminishing dandruff flakes. Or peanut oil and lemon juice
work well, say dermatologists. First, massage the scalp
with warm peanut oil, then apply fresh lemon juice. Leave
on a few minutes, then shampoo as usual.

Exercises for Stimulating the Scalp and Growing New Hair

1. Bend from the waist with the head toward the floor. With a natural bristle brush or widespread nylon bristles with protective knobs, brush the hair floorward. Take the stroke from the root of the hair along the scalp to the ends of the hair. The entire scalp and hair should feel the massage, the stimulation, the tugging.

2. Then, using the brush bristles, "scrub" the scalp. Apply the brush to an area of the scalp and scrub or massage — lift the brush and apply to another area until you have stimulated the complete scalp, especially across the top, the temples and the crown. Be sure you are bending from the waist so fresh blood may flood the cells. Instead of the brush, you may wish to use a small plastic hair massager with plastic teeth and a strap that fits over the back of the hand. It will bring a rapid flow of blood to the scalp and, at the same time, slough off dandruff flakes and loosen much clogging debris.

3. Now discard the brush. Using both hands, massage the scalp with the fingertips. Then grasp handfuls of hair and, still bending, pull the hair toward the floor. Pull and tug the hair all over the head. This pulling technique, especially with the head down and the blood flowing into the tissues of the scalp, lifts the scalp free of the skull. As the roots of the hairs are lifted, fresh blood flows into the bulb, dissolving any stagnated deposits of dirt, pollution, cholesterol, grime and oil. These obstacles, which cut off and block the flow of blood and pranic life force to the hair follicles, are briefly removed. So tug and hold, tug and hold, until the entire head of hair is stimulated. If you have already lost too much hair to pull vigorously across

the front and crown, then pinch up the scalp itself between the hands and between the thumb and forefinger, lifting small portions from the skull. Soon you may have new hair to lift.

4. Still bending from the waist, now place your hands over the frontal temple area of the scalp and lock your fingers. Applying pressure to the scalp, move it from side to side; then front to back. A tight scalp is a major cause of hair loss. It must be loosened. Now move the hands to the crown of the head, lock the fingers, apply pressure and move the scalp again — from side to side and from front to back. Continue this scalp loosening procedure, covering the entire head — then repeat it, flexing the scalp muscles until they move easily upon the frame of the skull. These scalp muscles must be flexed and massaged every single day, so that a rich supply of blood and pranic life force may reach the blocked blood vessels which feed the hair. If women wish to use the brush to "back comb" or "tease" the hair for fullness and fluffiness, it is best done while bending over. The brush is far better than using the comb, which tightens the hair into knots when "teasing."

5. Now stand erect. Using a brush and comb, groom your hair for the day. Avoid metal or fine combs. Choose one of hard rubber with smooth blunt-ended teeth. Or choose a plastic "spade" type comb with long far-apart teeth. It "fluffs" hair beautifully.

What are you accomplishing? Obviously you are stimulating the scalp, improving circulation, and removing dead hairs, all extremely important and necessary for continued hair health. The brushing and pulling will remove dead hairs, opening the way for the growth of new hairs as your scalp improves in circulation. So, in the beginning, if you seem to be losing too much hair, don't let this deter you. The dead hairs *must* be removed. As the pulling continues, when separation between scalp and skull occurs, circulation is stimulated, the blood rushes into every cell and gland, distributing necessary nutrients.

As for the muscle flexing, you are restoring the galea membrane to normalcy. Covering the crown of the head in both men and women is a thin sheet-like tendonous membrane called the *galea*. The galea is a muscle tying together the frontal muscle of the forehead and the occipital muscle at the back of the head. The galea membrane frequently thickens and becomes enlarged, creating a pressure and tension on the scalp, closing off the supply of blood through the small blood capillaries located just above the galea. It is this blood supply which feeds the hair follicles with the nutrients upon which the hair depends for growth.

The reason men become bald more frequently than women may be because the galea thickens in the male, whereas in the female it usually remains thin and elastic. This may be because women have a special chromosome which usually prevents baldness. An excessive flow of male hormone, testosterone, could be responsible for the thickening of the membrane. To restore the membrane to normal, practice the steps just given, especially the hair pulling and the muscle-flexing with the locked fingers. The membrane must be massaged, stretched and kept loose on the skull.

Aids to Overcoming Baldness

1. To avoid losing hair, to overcome dandruff, or if you just desire healthier, thicker hair, massage the scalp at bedtime with the following "old home remedy": to equal parts of castor oil and kerosene add one tablespoon of garlic

juice and mix well. After gently massaging the scalp allow
it to remain overnight. Or mix kerosene with the yolk of
an egg and apply to the scalp gently. Do not massage vigorously since the kerosene will cause a burning sensation.
Shampoo in the morning.

2. Mix the yolk of an egg, one or two tablespoons of olive
oil and two ounces of camomile tea. Massage every evening
until your hair begins to respond. Shampoo in the morning.

3. Add yeast and kelp tablets to your diet.

4. Swim in the ocean when possible. Ocean swimming
is renowned as an excellent treatment for the hair, if you
do not dry the hair afterward in full sunlight. The hair
should be dried in the shade giving the minerals and salts
in the ocean water an opportunity to slowly become
absorbed into the scalp and hair follicles. After thoroughly
dried, shampoo to remove the excessive salt from the hair.

5. Unless you have a heart problem, perform the yogic
headstand, which will thin the thickening galea membrane
and stimulate the scalp. The pressure will aid in dissolving accumulated salt crystals. Or, if the headstand is too
difficult, perform the half headstand. Simply place the top
of the head on the floor (or pad) and, with the feet flat on
the floor, raise the buttocks into the air.

6. Consider a slant board, which reverses the pull of
gravity upon the bloodstream. Nourishing blood flowing
from the heart feeds the hair and brain cells. If the bloodstream and the arteries are clogged when you are in your
normally upright position, it is doubtful whether the hair
receives its full supply of life giving blood, which must flow
"uphill." Lying on a slant board allows direct passage to
the brain and scalp, feeding the hair its needed nutrients.
If time is your problem, "slant" while watching TV.

7. Do be aware of the herb jojoba (pronounced ho-ho-ba) now being used to restore hair loss. Its most popular use is as a shampoo combined with applications of the jojoba oil directly to the scalp. Jojoba is a desert plant, bearing beans from which the precious oil is extracted. The product is available at most health stores. Jojoba oil removes encrusted sebum. Used as a shampoo it seals hair follicles against the damages of pollution, harsh chemicals, the heat of dryers, and the deadly rays of the sun.

8. Do have your doctor check for a thyroid deficiency. Low thyroid activity frequently results in hair loss. If your thyroid tests low, consider thyroid supplements from your health store rather than synthetic from your doctor. Also consider using a bar magnet over the gland to stimulate it. Order from Bio Health Enterprises, Inc. (See last chapter for address.) Ask for explicit instructions for stimulating a sluggish thyroid.

To test the thyroid at home, place a thermometer on your nightstand within easy reach. When you first waken, before stirring, place the thermometer under your arm pit. If your temperature reads low, you need thyroid therapy. I use a thermometer that "beeps" when the reading is ready. See my book, *The You Book: A Treasury of Health and Healing* for full details.

Beauty Treatment for the Hair

You may wish to try any of the following suggestions, all of which are most excellent to aid in conditioning and beautifying the hair. Some have been recognized as aiding baldness. All have been recognized as excellent to improve dryness, split ends, unnatural bleaching and to remove toxic conditions from the hair.

1. Combine an egg yolk with one-half cup of plain yogurt, apply to hair and soak from 10 to 30 minutes. Shampoo with warm water, not hot, and use a natural herbal shampoo.

2. Be aware of your *hair brush*. Once we believed a tightly packed bristle brush was superior, but we know now it isn't true. A brush with tightly packed bristles will not reach into "hair midst." It will tear hair out at the roots. It will split and damage any weak hairs. Available now are brushes with round heads, making it possible to reach the scalp for stimulation. The bristles will be spaced and have rounded tips to protect hair cuticles. Available now are brushes with wooden bristles. I ordered mine through a mail order catalog named Hoffritz (address in Chapter 10).

3. Your *comb* should be of heavy hard rubber with wide teeth. They are often available through your beauty operator. Use a hot comb only when vitally necessary. The same applies to curling irons, being sure yours has a teflon coating and thermostat.

4. Use heated curlers for natural effect occasionally, but not constantly. Too drying.

5. Do inquire about an all night permanent called an air ionizing wave which is used on delicate and very fine hair. I recently had one and I am very pleased with the results. If you live in the Southern California area, you can call Nelda Puopolo (address in Chapter 10).

6. Herbs have long been recognized as excellent hair beautifiers. Basically they are made into a tea and are used to clear dandruff, to add body, to lighten blond hair or darken brunette hair, to prevent baldness, to bring out luster, to condition damaged hair. For instance, elder flowers, lime flowers or nettles are excellent added to shampoo water. Parsley tea rubbed into the hair and scalp twice a

week will aid in clearing dandruff, while rosemary, added to the rinse water or poured over towel-dried hair, not only makes the hair fragrant but darkens dark hair. Camomile will lighten blond hair. Nettle helps restore natural color to gray hair. Bee pollen taken internally helps the hair keep its color.

Care of the Hair

1. Hair grows approximately one inch every six weeks. Its growth is more rapid in summer than in winter. And if one chooses to cut the hair at a propitious "moon" sign, the hair will grow either faster or more slowly depending upon the status of the moon at the time of cutting. According to certain astrologers, if you cut your hair when the moon is decreasing in light, from full moon to new moon, it will grow slowly. If you want it to grow faster, then cut it when the moon is increasing in light — from new to full. Have the hair trimmed often to remove split ends.

2. Once a week warm two tablespoons of cold pressed almond oil and massage into the scalp. Wrap the head in hot towels or cover with a plastic shower cap.

3. If possible, don't comb or brush hair while wet. The outer layer is soft and pliable, making it vulnerable to considerable breakage and damage. When possible, women should avoid rolling hair when it is wet. Wet hair stretches and, as it dries, it contracts. The tightly stretched hair is then vulnerable to considerable stress, resulting in breakage and damage. To repeat, roll the hair when almost dry, then spray it lightly preferably with rain water. This way the hair will only be damp when rolled, resulting in a prettier, more natural curl.

4. To "set" hair, use a flaxseed solution. Simply add flaxseed to a pan of water and bring to a boil. Strain and spray on hair before, during or after rolling.

5. Occasionally use a flat beer on your hair as a setting lotion. It adds body. Spray it on damp hair from a mist-spray bottle, very lightly. Too much creates a "gummy" appearance. And it must be flat so that undesirable chemicals in it have dissipated.

6. In cold winter weather wear a covering on your hair. Blasts of cold air dry and split hair. Do keep a humidifier in your home, especially in the bedroom for moisture in the hair as well as your skin.

7. There are various ways to protect your hair from the many summer activities the masses enjoy. First, the swimming pool. Chlorine in the water can dry and split the ends of your hair. Coat your hair with a protein moisturizer or protein pack before entering the pool. To prevent sun and water damage, consider applying a twenty minute deep conditioning treatment before entering the pool. Or use the Oak Bark Shampoo I've told you about and avoid the need of a conditioner. Always wear a bathing cap with your hair tucked safely inside. Always shower and shampoo your hair immediately after swimming. Ultraviolet rays can also damage your hair. Always wear a covering when exposed to the summer sun, or use an umbrella.

8. Apply shampoo only once unless your hair has been exposed to unusual dirt or dust. Habitually "soaping" twice could strip the hair of all natural oils, especially if done daily. Always apply an herbal protein conditioner unless you are using Fanie's Oak Bark Shampoo.

9. Use hair sprays only when absolutely necessary. Do read the labels and select the most natural product possible. And do brush it out as soon as possible. Its effect is

deadly, not only on the hair shaft, but in the lungs. Don't spray or use mousse except on special occasions. Constant use destroys the life force in the hair. Try your health store for the most natural and safe hair spray.

10. Be aware that you will experience the greatest hair loss in November, the least in May. Any time you lose more than a hundred hairs a day in your comb or brush, take action. Something is wrong. You may want to cancel all perms, all colorings and begin a program of hair health treatments. Change your hair style if you've drawn it tight. Loosen it and give it a chance to flow, in every possible way.

11. Avoid smoke-filled areas when possible. Nicotine smoke is deadly, not only for *you* but for your hair. When exposed, shampoo as soon as possible.

12. To give your hair fullness, brush or blow-dry while bending over. Then tease lightly with your hair brush. Standing erect, fluff out with your hands or special plastic fluffing comb.

13. Always check the profile of your hair to make sure the sides look as good as the front.

Hair Restoration

Avocado Treatment — The following is sworn to be a tried and true method of not only restoring hair and preventing the loss of hair but of restoring color to gray hair: Secure an avocado, tree ripened if possible. Place it in an obscure place to ripen further. Allow it to remain there, untouched, until it becomes black and mushy. Touching will cause a growth of fungus on the fruit. When it is black and mushy, shampoo and towel dry your hair, just blotting the excess water. Apply the avocado. After apply-

ing, massage with the fingertips from the ears upward. It
can remain anywhere from five minutes to all day, even
overnight, but 30 minutes is ideal. Rinse with warm
water. The hair will have been fed with pure protein and
the finest natural oils, which combat encrusted sebum oil.
Shampoo anywhere from an hour to a day later, for a final
removing of the remaining avocado oil. This excellent
treatment may be repeated again at your convenience.
Each time it is applied, expect a more luxuriant head of
hair — and a possible return to its natural color for gray-
ing hair. So say those recommending this treatment.

Fanie's Hair Treatment — You've already read of
Fanie's Oak Bark Hair Treatment which, used once a
week, has been known to grow hair. You apply some of the
totally natural herbal brown liquid to dry hair, spray a bit
of water to slightly liquefy it, cover the head with a plastic
shower cap for twenty minutes for heat, then apply water
for shampooing. On other days, you use Fanie's regular
Oak Bark Shampoo. I never use anything else. My thinning hair certainly has responded well to this treatment.
Order from Fanie's distributors. (addresses in last chapter).

Gerovital — To repeat, tablets of a "youth" product
called Gerovital (GH3) may help the hair growth and prevent baldness. It certainly has helped my hair. I truly
believe it retains the color, too. For years I have used both
injections and tablets of Gerovital, obtained from Roma-
nia. It contains procaine and para-aminobenzoic acid. My
hair has never turned totally gray. It has remained dark
brown. This amazing GH3 (Gerovital) formula has, I
believe, also helped me retain a measure of youthfulness.
(I am now over seventy years of age.) Gerovital tablets are
now available from many sources. But if you are unable

to find them, write to Valjean McGinty (address elsewhere). Its formula of procaine and para-aminobenzoic acid also aids in destroying hardened sebum, resulting in the restoration of hair.

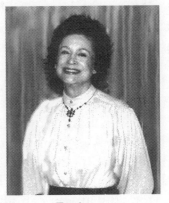

Earlyne

Honey and Onions — A book titled *Primitive Remedies*, written by Rev. John Wesley, founder of the Methodist Church over 200 years ago, has just been reissued by Woodbridge. Wesley says you can cure baldness by rubbing the scalp with honey and onions. He also says you can rub warts away with radishes. Maybe so! Try it. At least his remedies were "natural" and free of toxic chemicals.

KaminoMoto Scalp Energizer and Shampoo — is reputed to truly restore hair growth. Its major ingredient is a very rare herbal oil that comes from Japan and Formosa. The oil is extracted from the Japanese Kinoki tree. The manufacturers say the oil dissolves the encrusted sebum in the follicles of the hair and kills the bacteria resulting from the buildup of sebum. Once the bacteria is destroyed and the sebum deep in the follicles has been dissolved, hair growth follows naturally. The user is warned not to expect rapid results. If not available from your health store, order from Swanson's Health Products (address in Chapter 10). It's for both men and women. It's almost nonoily and dries quickly. I often massage it on my hair, then roll it for overnight. I like it because it doesn't require a daily shampoo.

Minoxidil — a high blood pressure drug released through Upjohn Company of Kalamazoo, Michigan, and presently advertised as a hair restorer, certainly is not the answer for everyone. Dr. Paul Lazer, former chairman of the American Medical Association's Committee on Cutaneous Health and Cosmetics, said statistics show it results in hair growth in about one in ten users. Even then, it takes from three to six months to obtain results. Because of its cost, its use is prohibitive for most. Once the user stops its use, the hair falls again. So says Dr. Lazer. But if you can afford it, it's worth considering.

Last minute warning! — just as these writings were going to press, an article arrived regarding Minoxidil. Although it certainly makes hair grow, it may pose serious health threats for older men. It contains a solution called *Rogaine* which produces fluid retention and increases the heart beat. Although not enough Minoxidil is absorbed through the scalp to cause serious reactions on most users, there are those who have a higher absorption rate than others. Such an absorption could be serious for those with high blood pressure, coronary heart disease or congestive heart failure, especially if they are on other medication. Physicians are being urged to advise users of Minoxidil (Rogaine) to look for warning signs, such as swelling. Potential users should first have a physical exam, then be monitored regularly to note any change for the worse. Its manufacturer, the Upjohn Company, explains that Minoxidil (Rogaine) is a treatment, not a cure. If the drug is stopped, the new hair will fall out within six months.

Minoxidil Plus Retin-A — Dr. Nia Terezakis of Tulane University and Dr. Jack Jaffe, the medical director of Physicians Hair Center at Boston, have released a report that the combination of Minoxidil plus Retin-A is proving extremely effective in conquering baldness — far more than Minoxidil alone. If interested you may want your doctor to contact these sources for full details.

New Genesis Hair Lotion — is a product developed in Canada. Dermatologists at Toronto General Hospital report that 77% of participating users showed "a significant and observable" increase in permanent hair restoration. The Canadian Health Protection Branch, Canada's equivalent of our FDA, has approved the product. I'm not familiar with its formula so cannot comment as to its contents. But it seems worth a try.

Omexin Active Treatment — The manufacturers of this new product swear it will cause the hair to grow. It contains *Zomexin*, a natural fatty compound called a lipid. It is not a drug. If you are interested in more information, call the manufacturer's toll-free at 1-800-666-3946. Several users have contacted me to report incredible results — usually within thirty to sixty days.

Polysorbate — We have said that too much male hormone testosterone, settling on the scalp, can block the flow of blood and disrupt the natural functioning of the hair follicles. Scientists, using an emulsifier called polysorbate to clean the scalps of skin cancer patients, discovered their patients were growing hair. Available on the market are several products containing polysorbate, guaranteed to grow hair. Investigate. Again, check with your doctor first.

Rum — Yes, rum! Jamaican rum is said to be a sure cure for baldness. The Jamaican men rub 126 proof rum into their scalps and visitors to the island say the men there have beautiful hair. Apparently it does more than just grow hair; it grows healthy hair.

Something New Under the (China) Sun — I've just read a report of a struggling country physician in the remote mountain area of Zhezian, China, who is said to have invented a cure for baldness in the 1970s. He was experimenting with a combination of oils and local herbs, such as ginseng, Chinese Angelica, dried ginger, walnut meat, safflower and alcohol. His concoction was so successful it's now becoming famous. If you're interested contact Dr. Zhao Zhangguang, c/o Bureau of Civil Affairs, Beijing People's Government, Beijing, People's Republic of China. After a couple of months use, results are said to be astounding. Well, we well know the power of ginseng and the other herbs. Why not write to secure a supply and try it — with your doctor's consent, of course. American pharmaceuticals will sooner or later bring it into our country. If they do, let's hope they won't add a bunch of chemicals so they can sell it as an expensive drug!

Vodka Cocktail — Beauty consultant-biochemist, Riquette Hoffstein, says she has developed a deep cleansing formula that unclogs the pores of the scalp and stimulates new hair growth. Ingredients: 1/4 cup of vodka, 10 aspirins, 2 Alka Seltzer tablets, 1 tsp. cayenne pepper and 2 tsp. of Hoffstein's "Scalp Shampoo." With a soft toothbrush, apply the cocktail to your scalp using a gentle, circular motion until your head is covered. Massage the remaining mixture in to dissolve any oily residue. Apply once a week.

To make the Scalp Shampoo, set aside 1 tbsp. crushed basil leaves; 1 tbsp. lavender flowers; 1 tbsp. rosemary leaves. Add them to 3 cups boiling water and then remove from heat. Next, strain into 1/2 cup of liquid castile soap. Daily shampooing is recommended. Since Fanie's Oak Bark Shampoo already contains many herbs, if you're too busy to concoct this shampoo, why not use Fanie's daily and the special cocktail formula once a week?

Now, having written a whole chapter concerning the hair and its restoration, let me say how I really feel, personally, about baldness. *I think bald is beautiful!* Of course, it's nice if hair can be saved but, if it can't, why worry unduly? It's not worth emotional stress and struggle. It's far more important to be happy. Tension over baldness means a tight scalp. So live as relaxed as possible. Brush often, massage often — and laugh much. Live healthy and holy. Remember always that your heavenly crown is more important than your crowning glory — the hair.

For Beautiful Hands

Pour a teaspoon of raw whole milk into a palm and massage your hands with it until it is absorbed. Follow with lemon juice or rubbing the hands with a peel of lemon. Allow it to dry. This is particularly effective at bedtime, especially if you wear cotton cosmetic gloves to bed, available at drug stores. Try applying mayonnaise at bedtime, also — and, again, use cotton gloves.

Beautiful Nails — The nails require attention, but the manicure need not be arduous. Do use a diamond steel nail file for filing instead of an emery board. Don't saw back and forth. File gently in one direction. File the nails with square corners. Nails filed in the corners tend to split and break. If there is polish to remove, do use an oil-based product. And wash off the polish remover immediately, since it will dry and corrode the nail if left on. Then soak a few minutes in half and half oil and warm water. It softens the cuticle. Apply a good oil to the nails, preferably olive or almond to which vitamin E oil has been added. Push back the cuticles with a Q-Tip or orangewood stick, aided by a soft washcloth. But do not unduly disturb the cuticle. It will only cause it to split and become tough. Split cuticles are the bane of beautiful hands. The purpose of the cuticle is to protect the nail bed against infection. Never cut it, except to snip off the tip where hangnails may appear. Try buffing your nails until they shine. Buffing brings blood to the nail bed and beauty to the nail itself.

Nail Polish — Avoid colored nail polish as much as possible. It contains butyl acetate, nitrocellulose, ethyl acetate, toluene, dibutyl phthalate, alkyl ester, dyes, glycol derivatives, gums, hydrocarbons both aromatic and aliphatic, formaldehyde resin, ketones, lakes (colorings) and phosphoric acid. The colorings and dyes usually include D and C Red Nos. 6, 7, 19, 31, 34 and Yellow No. 5. Allergies to these ingredients include skin rashes, irritation of the fingernail tissues, nails permanently stained black, fungus, discolored nails, splitting nails and nausea. *All* DC colors are derivatives of coal tar, a known carcinogen. If used constantly, nail polish dyes could be absorbed into the skin and thus into the system, resulting either in cancer or unpleasant reactions of allergy, the sources usually unknown to the victim. These dyes have now been removed from food since they are recognized causes of cancer. Why not wear only a clear colorless polish and use a nail whitener pencil under the nails? It's beautiful. And much more safe. To whiten further under the nails, use a cotton tipped applicator dipped in hydrogen peroxide for bleaching. If you must use polish, first apply a base clear undercoat.

Never, never apply fake nails unless an important engagement is pending and one of yours *must* be repaired. Acrylic nails not only look fake, but they can cause appalling damage to your nails — even the glue used is dangerous. Infections, fungus, the permanent loss of a nail could result.

Avoid most nail-hardening products. They contain harmful chemicals, especially formaldehyde. A few are natural protein-based, but be cautious. Consider *Fanie's Instant Nail Hardener* which contains keratin and sulfur, two of the components within the nail itself. It contains no harmful drugs or chemical stimulants. Or apply *Fanie's Anti-Fungus Thymolize*. It contains thymol iodide and potassium iodide, excellent for nail growth and for healing nail fungus. Also take Silica Herb tablets (Horsetail) daily which greatly help both nails and hair.

Avoid exposing the hands to water as much as possible. Do use rubber gloves. While watching television, apply olive oil to the nails nightly, massaging into the cuticles. Result: fantastic nails. Some prefer a mixture of castor oil and white iodine. Or apply Fanie's Nail Hardener or Thymolize.

Setting Nail Polish — If you insist on wearing polish, to harden the polish of a fresh manicure plunge the fingertips into a bowl of ice water. Polish hardens immediately with a clear finish. Or brush your nails with a vegetable oil, such as safflower, olive, etc. Polish dries instantly.

Fingernails and Health — In many of my previous writings, I've told you about dear old Dr. Som, the naturopath who taught me so much about vegetarianism and well-being. He said each time a new patient came to him he first looked at the hands, and especially the fingernails. He said the fingernails were a positive gauge to the health of the body. He studied the nails either under the sunlight or under a strong artificial light and always after the nail polish was removed. Since then many doctor friends have corroborated his statements.

Dr. Som said that if the nails were in poor health, the hair and joints would also be dry and brittle. The system needs oiling (flaxseed oil? — cod liver oil?). Emotions affect the hair and nails immensely. Thick nails indicate poor circulation. White spots are no cause for alarm since they are simply bruises. But pale fingernails often indicate anemia or lack of iron. When the nails turn yellow it may be a sign of kidney problems. Ridges on the nails could also be connected with kidney problems. Blisters on fingertips could signal a serious circulation problem. Small sores, scleroderma. If a blue color appears at the base of the nail it could mean you have silver in your system. Consider doing something about the silver-mercury fillings in your teeth. Inflamed skin around the nails could signal diabetes. Red around the base of the nail may relate to a heart problem. Nails that simply keep splitting and breaking may be a symptom of lack of silica which is available at your health store. Iron deficiency could cause the nails to dip inward causing them to be called spoon nails. So said Dr. Som.

Chapter Seven

The Tooth — and Nothing but the Tooth

Your teeth really should last a lifetime if you take good care of them. Do consider brushing with salt, soda, myrrh and oak bark powder, described later. Periodontal disease accounts for 70% of tooth loss, so don't forget to floss daily and have your teeth cleaned every six months. It's good, too, to use a Water Pik daily to remove food and to stimulate the gums.

Plaque is a sticky film loaded with bacteria that irritates the gums. It can eventually destroy the bone supporting the teeth. Left untreated, teeth can loosen and fall out. Trouble is, it can progress with no discomfort until it reaches advanced stages. In the beginning it appears as gingivitis (inflammation of the gums) and, if not checked, progresses to periodontal disease. Bleeding gums signal a problem.

Gum Disease — The leading culprit for the loss of teeth is gum disease, not tooth decay. Gum disease begins with the buildup of bacteria in the gap between the teeth and gums. Such bacteria is extremely toxic and irritates the gum tissue, causing inflammation. If the bacteria is not removed, it seeps further under the gums, eventually causing pockets of infection to form, resulting in bleeding, swelling and bad breath. It also causes the gums to recede from the teeth which can loosen them. If you are being treated for gum disease, a new test helps to check whether a patient's gums have been healed. It's called DNDX. The test costs between $75 and $125. Do ask your dentist for details.

Brush after each intake of food, if possible — at least twice a day. Have a toothbrush at your place of employment. Rinse twice a day with an antibacterial mouthwash, such as *Plax* or *Listerine*. They loosen plaque. Use just before brushing. Don't hesitate to use a toothpick or *Stimudents* gently around your teeth. Do rinse your mouth following a glass of wine, beer or alcoholic beverage. They can eat away at fillings, bondings, some types of crowns and veneers. This is also true of all sweets. Avoid diet sodas. They can destroy tooth enamel, even though they are sugarless. They contain destructive acid, especially those containing "fruit" juices.

To protect your teeth from acid damage during sleep, my dentist suggested applying thick *Milk of Magnesia* at bedtime. Pour off most of the liquid which rises to the top and use the creamy substance. With your finger, apply the Milk to your gums. Or take a mouthful and swish it through the teeth, but don't swallow it. It contains aluminum. Its residue will coat the teeth and gums with a protective alkaline cover, shielding them from the mouth acids which accumulate while sleeping.

If you suffer from bacterial endocarditis, congenital

heart abnormalities, any heart valve disorder, or if you have undergone heart valve surgery, ask your doctor to give you an antibiotic to destroy infection one hour before any dental work which could cause bleeding. When mouth bacteria enters the bloodstream it could cause fever, chills, rapid destruction of a heart valve and heart failure, says the American Heart Association.

Erosion of tooth enamel can occur through your daily swim, due to exposure to acid in chlorinated pool water. The acid softens tooth enamel, causing it to wear down quickly and making teeth extremely sensitive to heat and cold. Do rinse your mouth with a solution of water and baking soda before and after the swim to neutralize the acid. Or use the Milk of Magnesia just suggested. If damage has already been done, seek at your health store for minerals and trace minerals to replace the lost minerals in your teeth.

Easing Toothache — Until you can get to a dentist, ease a toothache by applying ice to the web of skin between your thumb and index finger. Hold in place by a gauze bandage for up to seven minutes, or until the area feels totally numb. Apply the ice to the hand on the same side as the toothache.

Soak a wad of pure cotton in oil of cloves and hold it on an aching tooth. Purchase the oil at a drug store. For a cracked tooth or loose filling, again the oil of cloves. Avoid sweets, hot food and crunchy food. Occasionally rinse with part water and part hydrogen peroxide.

For bleeding gums, rinse your mouth often with warm salt water. Use warm salt water in your Water Pik to heal and firm the gums, and to destroy embedded bacteria and infections.

Toothpaste or Powder — Nothing is more controversial than fluoride toothpaste. Those expounding its benefits claim that such toothpaste is effective in reducing the incidence of tooth decay. Those opposed voice dire warnings as to its potential accumulative danger. There are leading authorities on both sides. Most dental paste or powder uses abrasives for maximum cleaning efficiency, which includes calcium carbonate, dibasic calcium phosphate, dehydrate anhydrous, tricalcium phosphate, calcium pyrophosphate, insoluble sodium metaphosphate and hydrated alumina. These substances are absorbed into the body through osmosis and the saliva. What potential dangers they present are at the present unknown.

My dentist — one of the finest in Southern California — is vociferously opposed to fluoride toothpaste. His reasons are too numerous to include here. He suggests the use of simple baking soda and fine salt as a tooth powder. Salt and soda was our dentifrice when I was a child growing up at home — and my mother often added charcoal powder. She prepared the mixture herself. All five of her children had beautiful white teeth. I don't know where she got her information, perhaps psychically. I still use salt and soda. The salt I use is either *Real Salt* from my health store, or salt from the Dews Company (address elsewhere). But I also add powdered myrrh and oak bark powder from the health store, equal amounts of all four. I keep my powder mixture in a small open container with a small container of hydrogen peroxide nearby. I first wet my brush with faucet water, then dip it in the hydrogen peroxide, then into the powder. I use Plax and I brush often, even after snacks, and I floss nightly, usually using *Superfloss*. If you'd like to add charcoal to your salt and soda mixture, it's available as capsules at your health store. Just open the capsules and add the charcoal powder. If charcoal is used in most water purifiers, it must be qualified to destroy bacteria in the mouth.

You may prefer *Peelu* toothpaste or tooth powder, available at health stores. Peelu contains fibers which the manufacturers claim effectively removes plaque. The toothpaste and powder contain no harsh abrasives as is usually found in commercial powders and pastes. Peelu products are made from the peelu tree which contains several natural chemicals that aid in the removal of plaque, one of which is natural chloride. It also contains substances which act as natural antibiotics, reducing the spread of plaque-building bacteria. The peelu tree also contains sulfur compounds which provide antibacterial effects.

Silver Dental Fillings — Much is now said and written about the continued use of silver fillings in teeth. The controversy concerning their use has split the dental industry, the minority being those dentists who are becoming aware of their potential danger and who now refuse to use such material. They well know that "silver" isn't silver in the material they receive from their laboratories. It's made of alloys. The silver alloy contains mercury, and could contain nickel and beryllium. All are toxic, but mercury is the chief culprit in silver amalgams. Ask for a composite or gold rather than a silver filling.

But often you do not avoid harm by asking for gold fillings. Alas, dental "gold" is not gold, though the dentist has paid the exorbitant fee for your filling and has passed the price on to you. The gold has been found to be from 2% to 80% pure. Its "fillers" are nickel and beryllium. Both are extremely toxic. To be sure you aren't allergic to the gold of your intended filling, have your dentist send you with a sample to a dental specialist who possesses a Voll machine. Tests on such a machine could alert you to your reaction to the chosen gold. My specialist did even better. Using a Voll machine, he tested me on 12 varieties of gold, finding out that three were deadly to me. So we chose a "safe" gold. It may not have been totally pure, but at least we knew that whatever metal was added was safe for me. You may prefer a polymer-ceramic composite and avoid all metal, even gold. But have it, too, tested on a Voll machine.

The danger of silver fillings, again, is the deadly mercury. It's not supposed to leak into the bloodstream and the immune systems but tests have proven conclusively that it does. The mysterious diseases that go into remission after the silver fillings are removed are too numerous to mention. For full details about the "silver" controversy, see *The You Book: A Treasury of Health and Healing*.

Herbal Gum Massage — Edgar Cayce recommended salt and soda as a dentifrice for those with bleeding gums and loose teeth. He also recommended the use of an herbal solution called *Peri-dent* to massage the gums or to use as a mouthwash. It contains purified water, prickly ash bark, sodium chloride, calcium chloride, iodine, grain alcohol and peppermint oil. It's available from wherever Cayce products are sold. So is a salt and soda preparation. I order from Cayce Corner, A.R.E. Clinic in Phoenix, Arizona (address elsewhere), established by Drs. Gladys and William McGarey.

Computers and Teeth — If you ever need crowns on your teeth, you'll be happy to know there is now a computer program that translates special photographs into computer images — then converts the image into exact measurements for shaping a new crown.

Teeth Grinding — The Academy of General Dentistry reports that people who sleep on their side or stomach are more apt to grind their teeth during sleep. Side sleepers wake with jaw pain. Stomach sleepers grind even more. They say the nongrinders are those who sleep on the back with a good support to the neck and with knee support. Gritting the teeth can be extremely serious. It's done mostly at night, when one is asleep and unaware. The constant gnashing can grind down the teeth, loosen them, tire the chewing muscles, and cause pain at the jaw joint just in front of the ears. Do ask your dentist regarding a "bite" plate at night. It's a device to cushion the teeth to save them further grinding. He may prescribe a splint to protect from further damage.

Continued stress could cause trench mouth, a bacterial infection of the gums. Stress increases the outflow of cortisal from the adrenals, which could impair the immune system. Failure of the body to dispose of the bacteria, due to too much cortisal, could result in trench mouth. Do consult your dentist in case of grinding teeth. Also be aware of your sleeping pillow. You need one that has a special shape, like a "chiropractor's" pillow, which I've mentioned previously. Again, for much more information and guidance concerning teeth, see *The You Book*.

Chapter Eight

Special Techniques for Rejuvenation

For a Beautiful Posture — View yourself nude in a full- length mirror. Do the shoulders slouch? Does your head droop forward instead of aligning with the spine? Is one shoulder lower than the other? Do your toes turn outward in a duck walk? — or inward in pigeon-toed fashion? One overall exercise will aid all these faults.

Stand facing a corner of your room. Place the hands on opposite walls of the corner. Now let the body slant forward as you try to touch the corner with your nose. Keep the spine and knees straight. Inhale as you indraw the tummy muscles. Indraw the pelvis, raise the chin and the chest so that the spine is straight. Keep the feet flat on the floor and stretch the muscles at the back of the heels. The entire stance will improve. Exhale as you straighten. Repeat several times. Nothing is superior to walking with a book or heavy object on the head to correct the stance, to upraise the breasts, to straighten slumped shoulders, to correct the pigeon-duck walk. Try it!

For a Flat Tummy — Lie down on a bed or the floor on your back, or stand straight and tall with your back against a wall. Now pull in the stomach *hard*. Contract and tense every muscle. Lying down is preferable, but if you are against a wall, try to press the small of the spine against the wall, making a straight line of the spine. Hold the breath, the indrawn stomach muscles, and the tension, as long as comfortable. Slowly exhale and release the tension. Relax a moment, then repeat. Repeat at least three times, preferably more because each time the tension is performed, the stomach flattens more. It not only temporarily improves the appearance, but repeated and frequent performance will strengthen the stomach muscles and help to permanently flatten a paunchy abdomen. It is a marvelous isometric exercise, not for youth alone but for health. A heavy overweight abdomen could create strain on the lower back, causing back pain. It could also cause a hernia. Male readers should try this, too.

Another technique: stand with feet wide apart. Bend the knees enough to place the hands on the front of the thighs between knees and crotch, with the elbows out. Indraw the breath, creating an indrawn cavity in the midsection. Now, while holding the breath, pump the stomach muscle in and out. Exhale and relax. Repeat several times for a flattened tummy. Or inhale and exhale vigorously, tensing the stomach muscles while inhaling.

Sanford Bennett, back in 1917, taught that rubbing the stomach would reduce the abdomen. While still abed, upon waking, lie on your back and tense your stomach muscles by bending your knees and raising your head. Now start massaging your stomach with your right hand, covered with the left, making circular movements from the right side to the left — clockwise movements. Relax. Tense again, then begin rubbing downward as if washing clothes on a scrub board, using both or one hand. Relax, tense again and pound your stomach with your fists. Repeatedly, massage from right to left while tensing the muscles. This will not only reduce the stomach but will greatly improve elimination, while releasing pockets of toxic wastes. Its benefits are enormous.

Copper Bras for a Beautiful Bust? — Those Japanese! A Japanese naturopath has invented a copper bra which is worn for the purpose of increasing the size of breasts. And its wearers swear it works. We all know copper is renowned for its healing properties — for instance, copper bracelets worn to offset the pain of arthritis. This bra is made of copper mesh and is supposed to stimulate the growth of breasts. It is supposed to be marketed worldwide soon. So-o we'll see!

Deep Breathing for Relaxation and Beauty — You may not wish to perform the complete Yoga Breath so marvelous for the total being — but here is a modified version you can *easily* practice with little effort. Lie flat on your back. Inhale slowly through the nostrils, taking the breath all the way down to the abdomen. Concentrate on extending the stomach as far out as possible — a round mound of a tummy. Place a heavy book over the abdomen to aid in this technique if you wish. Hold the breath as long as comfortable. Then open and purse your lips. Exhale slowly, gradually indrawing the muscles of the abdomen until it is flat. Try to pull the abdomen up and in, forcing the exhaling air up into the chest and out of the body. Relax, then repeat as often as possible. Try this just before sleeping. You will sleep more relaxed. It may also induce sleep for the insomniac. Continued practice will result in better health, total relaxation when needed, a balanced flow of yin-yang pranic force throughout the body, a deeper sweeter voice, sparkling eyes, vibrant complexion, a flatter stomach and an increase in personal magnetism.

Arm Jogging — Whereas I do not approve of jogging, it's different with arm jogging. Jogging with the feet is very hard on the legs, ankles and knees — and the heart is put to great effort pumping the blood upward from the moving legs. But arm jogging is actually good for circulation. From the moving arms, blood flows downward from the heart, improving circulation throughout the body. Lying flat on your back, extend your arms back over your head. Now swing them forward to your sides, alternating the arms. Begin slowly and increase your jogging as you progress. Begin with ten arm flaps and increase as your muscles grow stronger. Now, still lying on your back, imagine there is a punching bag in front of you. Punch it vigorously. While standing, raise your arms to the side. Bring them together in front with a gentle slap, then raise them over your head and back to the sides. Repeat several times. Now, hum a little tune and keep time to the music with your arms as if you were conducting an orchestra. For that matter, turn on your favorite music station and dance with your whole body. It reduces and it exercises every muscle.

Strengthening the Legs — While sitting on the edge of your chair, lift your legs parallel to the floor and hold them for a few seconds. Then lower them slowly. Repeat, ten times. For even greater effect, drape a weight over each ankle or one ankle at a time, raising either both legs or one at a time. A bean bag or a thawed package of frozen vegetables will do the trick.

Let's Take a "Commercial" Break

Why not don your pajamas at the beginning of the evening and watch television in loose clothing? This will encourage you to perform several important exercises without actually leaving the television room. It is not the best time nor manner to perform exercises, to be sure, but since so many spend so much time before the tube to the neglect of bodily exercise, it is better that they be performed there than not at all. Instead of rushing to the refrigerator for that piece of cake or pie or potato chips, let's do something good for your body — let's exercise! Not only is this excellent therapy but you're apt to lose some weight also. Spread the exercises over several commercials. It's a good idea to buy an exercise pad or an old quilt at a thrift store, because some are practiced lying on the floor.

1. Sit upright in your chair and drop your head so your chin touches your chest. Stretch your neck forward. Then try to touch each shoulder with each ear, side-stretching your neck. Now, lift your head and stretch your neck, pretending you are attempting to reach the ceiling with your scalp. Hold the stretch a moment, then relax. Repeat several times.

2. Rotate the feet and ankles. Then apply the techniques for acupressure and reflexology, not only on the feet but all over the body. If you aren't familiar with acupressure points, buy a book which will enlighten you. If you have a vibrator, use it now, especially on the feet.

3. While sitting on a firm padded surface on the floor perform the spinal rock. Lock the arms or hands beneath the bent knees. Now leaning backwards, bring the knees with you as you rock back and forward again on the sacrum for a count of twenty. There is a device called the Abdo-

minizer which simulates this yogic exercise. Though not as effective as the spinal rock it may offer aid in accomplishing a similar purpose. (Address in Chapter 10).

4. Lying on the floor, grasp your right elbow with your left hand and your left elbow with your right hand. Inhale, tense every muscle of your body while gripping your arms tightly with each hand. Hold the breath for a long inhalation, then relax completely, exhaling deeply. Repeat several times.

5. Lying on the floor, draw your knees up to your chest and hug them with your arms. Raise your head and tense the entire body. Press your spine flat against the floor and hold tension as long as you can hold the breath. Then exhale and repeat. Several times.

6. Lie face down on the floor with an exercise pad or a quilt beneath you. Place a small cushion beneath the abdomen. Inhale fully only through abdominal muscles, pushing the abdominal muscles against the pillow. During the inhalation, arch the body with the arms and legs slightly lifted so that increased abdominal pressure will push against the pillow. Holding the breath, rock on the pillow with only the abdominal muscles supporting you. Hold for the count of five. Relax for the count of five and repeat three more times.

7. Lying on your back, draw one knee as close to the chest as possible. Place one hand on the knee and the other on the ankle. Press the raised ankle against the hand while the hand holds the ankle in place. Then try to straighten the leg as the hand on the knee holds it firmly in place. Then pull the leg firmly toward the chest. Release the leg and repeat the same with the other leg.

8. Stand erect, keeping your shoulders down and relaxed. Lift your left arm toward the front and rotate it

slowly backward making a complete circle. Allow it to perform full swings ten times. Then change arms and repeat
with the right arm.

9. Stand erect. Inhale deeply as you raise your arms
toward the ceiling and stretch — stretch — stretch. Now
fall over from the waist, rag doll fashion, allowing your
head and arms to dangle loosely. Let your arms gradually
begin to rotate in circles as you bounce the upper torso up
and down, gently flexing your spine, as your head hangs
downward. As you come up erect, inhale slowly and stretch
again. Fall over several times, exhaling and inhaling
deeply. You'll soon be able to touch the floor with your dan-
gling rotating hands.

10. If you have my *Book of Beginning Again* you may
want to perform the isometric (tension and relaxing) techniques offered there by Sanford Bennett.

11. If you are familiar with the yogic exercise called
Salutation to the Sun you may wish to perform it now.

12. This one requires a table so possibly cannot be performed while watching TV. Stand near a table, far enough
away so that while leaning forward there is a pull on the
calves of the legs. Slant the whole body forward, keeping
the knees straight. Grasp the edge of the table. Keep the
heels flat on the floor. Now step forward with one leg, bending the leg at the knee. Keep pressing forward until
pulling is felt in the ankle and calf of the back leg — the
extended leg. Now switch legs and repeat. Contracting
and relaxing the calf and ankle muscles helps to prevent
a buildup of inflamed calcium deposits in the heels.

13. Stand with one leg on top of a table. The leg should
be straight and the knee should not be bent. Lean the
upper body forward until tension is felt back of the thighs.
Use no force. Rock gently backward and forward, tensing

and relaxing the hamstring muscles. Repeat on the other leg.

Now, back to the T.V. movie! But, remember — television often subconsciously irritates. If you just push the "off" button and climb into bed you may have difficulty relaxing into sleep. So, when you're ready, turn the TV off and perform the following exercise and see if you don't have a more restful sleep.

Step to an open window and raise your arms directly in front of you, level with the shoulders. Inhale deeply as you swing your arms back as far as they will go, attempting to touch your hands behind you. Repeat the swinging of the arms from front to back for several deep breaths, then exhale vigorously and relax.

Now to bed — and sweet dreams.

Chapter Nine

Guidelines to
Keeping Young

The Ayurveda Approach — Out of India comes the Ayurveda (knowledge of life) approach to natural healing and rejuvenation techniques, said to be the oldest system of natural health care in the world. The Ayurveda system includes dietary guidance, herbal supplements, massage and meditation to aid in healing. Its advocates contend that disease is caused by improper diet, pollutants, stress, and the interruption of our natural cosmic body rhythms caused by unwise life-styles. The massage includes a body rub using warm sesame oil.

I feel sure Ayurveda *is* one of the oldest methodologies for healing, just now reappearing on the health scene. But we cannot discount our own "holistic" (or wholistic) approach, which is to treat the whole person, not simply to focus on a titled illness. I think our modern holistic movement may have surfaced simultaneously with the ancient Ayurveda system in our modern world. Ayurveda is superior when a medical doctor, with his knowledge of the latest medical approach, will include the entire natural Ayurvedic approach

under one roof — whereas in our holistic system, we poor
patients have to run hither and yon to find a holistic doctor,
a knowledgeable herbalist, a good dietitian, a fabulous
masseur or masseuse, healing through colored lights and
music, a homeopathic chiropractor or osteopath, a reflexol-
ogist, or an acupuncturist, in various locations. God bless
the day American clinics will embrace the entire holistic
concept in one location, with access to all methodologies for
the new age seeker of natural healing, including, too, the concept of Ayurveda.

The Ayurvedic approach is superior to our Western holistic approach, too, in that it concerns itself with the five elements of ether, fire, air, water, earth; the three bodily humors
(tridosha); the seven body tissues (dhatus); the three elimination issues: urine, stool and perspiration (malas); and the
trinity of humankind — the body, mind and spirit. Our
Western consciousness has not yet totally embraced the idea
of energy manifesting in the five basic elements — that is,
the concept of air, fire, water, earth and ether as they relate
to our five senses. Ayurveda teaches that ether relates to
hearing, air to touch, fire to vision, water to taste, and earth
to smell. And Ayurveda involves the individual in his/her
own healing and well-being, eventually evolving toward and
into cosmic consciousness. Let's hope that the dawning new
age will see these ancient concepts becoming integrated into
our medicine, our philosophy and our religion. To learn more
of this unique approach to youth and well-being, seek literature concerning Ayurveda at your metaphysical book store.

**"Will You Please Refrain from Smoking — I'm Aller-
gic"** — People who don't smoke are quite justified in asking
others not to smoke in their vicinity. Cigarette smoke in a
closed room concentrates nicotine and dust particles so dense
the nonsmoker inhales as much as a smoker inhales from

four or five cigarettes. Smoke from an idling cigarette contains almost twice the tar and nicotine of smoke inhaled by
the smoker — because the cigarette smoked by the smoker is
filtered. Thus the nonsmoker who is constantly exposed to
smoke from either idling or "active" cigarettes runs far more
risk of injury than the smoker! In a poorly ventilated smoke-
filled room, concentrations of carbon monoxide can easily
reach several hundred parts per million — a definite toxic
hazard for both smoker and nonsmoker. Many who suffer
from emphysema may be the victims of smoker's smoke.

One of the major problems I faced while leading tours of
travelers to mystical sites all over the world was that of sep-
arating the smokers from the nonsmokers on the buses. Both
had paid their fares and deserved consideration. But since
many nonsmokers experienced actual allergic reactions when
exposed to smoke we had no choice but to find a solution. We
placed all smokers on a bus all to themselves. When this
wasn't practical, we established the policy of stopping the bus
occasionally to allow all smokers to alight and smoke outside
the bus. So everyone was happy. The smoker has become very
aware of the effect his or her smoke has upon others, and is
usually considerate and understanding. It's hard for the
nonsmoker to be equally considerate, since few understand
the plight of the smoker who cannot smoke. But what is difficult for anyone to understand is why youngsters who know
the risks involved would ever begin such a habit in the first
place.

Youth and Factor Q-10 — What is Factor Q-10? It's an
enzyme, and it's essential for life. It's a chemical produced
in your own body. When your immune system fails to produce
sufficient quantities, disease occurs. And when the Q-10 factor falls even lower, death occurs — because it's the ultimate
chemical substance that gives life to every cell in the body.

Q-10 was first discovered in 1957 by Dr. Frederick L. Crane at Purdue University. He isolated the chemical from a bovine heart. Since then research has revealed its tremendous importance in relation to health. When the body fails to produce a high percentage all the organs slow down, the glands fail to distribute proper amounts of hormones, muscles lose tone and fail to function properly, memory fails, hair turns gray, wrinkles appear, energy levels drop, fat accumulates. Happily, Factor Q-10 is now available in capsule form at your health store. It comes in various potencies. If you can afford it, purchase the highest potency — 30 milligrams. It's called "the youth pill." And it lives up to its reputation.

Hyperbaric Oxygen Chamber — the hyperbaric chamber that I told you about in *The You Book: A Treasury of Health and Healing,* is finally being recognized by the medical profession en masse, as they are now being installed in hospitals throughout the country.

The chamber, which supplies pure oxygen to the occupant's bloodstream, is now being hailed as the closest thing on earth to the fountain of youth. It not only helps to speed healing of various afflictions such as severe burns and infections, but it also rejuvenates the body, restoring youth and vitality as well. To learn more about this amazing life-saving machine, see *The You Book: A Treasury of Health and Healing.*

Germanium and Youth — Germanium (Ge-132) is another blockbuster! Or age-buster! The wonders of germanium read like the heal-all tonic of the traveling medicine man of not so long ago — a tonic guaranteed to heal anything from ingrown toenails to bald heads. Well, just read all the benefits of germanium:

It utilizes oxygen, flooding the body with this life-saving substance without which the tissues and cells die — and the body. This vitalized oxygen feeds starved tissues, cells and organs. Oxygen-starved cells cannot resist invading bacteria. Result: candida, a fungal yeast which, once embedded, is a host to other disorders.

Germanium fights the invasion of cancer cells. Not only does it ease the pain of advanced cancer, but it has even been reported to heal cancer. Cancer cannot take root in oxygen-rich cells. It fights free radicals. It cures chronic arthritis. It aids in restoring sexual powers; it prevents miscarriages; it heals burns without scarring; it cures radiation aftereffects. It aids in circulatory disorders such as heart attack and stroke. It aids in healing hepatitis and cirrhosis of the liver. It stimulates the immune system to resist the effects of toxic mercury, cadmium and polychlorinated biphenyls (PCBs). It has been known to bring high blood pressure under control. It aids hearing problems and osteoporosis.

Combined with Suma, a Brazilian herb, it is even more powerful in rebuilding a depleted immune system. Garlic is rich in germanium. So is ginseng. If you can find a supplement which combines Suma and ginseng, buy it. It's a powerful source of activated germanium. Aloe vera also contains germanium. Or you could take simultaneously your Ge-132 capsule (germanium), your garlic capsule, your Suma capsule, your ginseng capsule, and your Q-10 capsule. Drink them down with an ounce of aloe vera gel added to your glass of water. What immune system wouldn't respond! Germanium, Suma and all the capsules mentioned are available at your health store.

Youth and Ginseng — Long known in the orient as a source of prolonging life and as a stimulant of sexual energies, we Westerners have joined in its praise. Wild Siberian ginseng also increases stamina, relieves stress, helps prevent respiratory diseases, and aids in high blood pressure and heart problems. It clearly has an effect on brain cells, restoring memory and improving concentration. The herb is filled with vitamins, minerals and amino acids. Could we hope to find more in anything the good doctor could prescribe?

Gerovital — Don't forget what has already been written about GH3. There is absolutely no question that its ingredients contribute to youth. Its use in the restoration of hair is renowned. So is its effectiveness in relieving pain and illness — and wellness *always* manifests youth. I myself am a living testimony of its long-range effect. Now, in my 70s, I am truly in better health than in my youthful years. Of course, I'm also a vegetarian, which without question has contributed to my longevity. And there are other factors I've written about in my other books — *The Book of Beginning Again, The Eyes Have It and The You Book: A Treasury of Health and Healing* . But still, Gerovital has played a major role in my life drama of keeping young. See the last chapter for where to order if you're interested.

Subliminal Methods for Youth and Beauty— Subliminal tapes are now available for most any purpose. But none may apply to your own personal needs. Why not make your own? True, it may not be subliminal, but it will be extremely effective. Use your own tape recorder, or borrow one from a friend. Focus on your own need, write out your own suggestions, and dictate your own tape. It's to be used to reach your subconscious mind. You can attain most any goal by reaching and persuading your subconscious mind to act as your ally, especially if instructions are in your own voice.

Let's say you want to lose weight. Work out your own affirmations, record them on your tape, and set up proper conditions for playing the tape — perhaps at night when you can sit in total darkness except for the light of a candle. It might help to place a mirror directly before you so that as you listen to the tape you can gaze deeply into your own eyes. With only the glow of a candle, play the tape over and over, affirming the loss of weight. If you cannot produce such a tape, then write out your affirmations and speak them orally as you sit in the quiet alone. You may wish to tape a picture of yourself at your very best on the door of your refrigerator for visual reinforcement to your subconscious mind. There are several herbal teas which can be effective during the weeks of your program. They are available at your health store. One is called "Slim Tea." Or write to Michael Tierra for his own special herbal formula for weight loss.

Dr. Dupote Samritvanitch of Bangkok, Thailand, says the best and most natural method of losing weight is to place a lettuce seed on the end of one finger and press it against the inside of the ear ten times before each meal. The seed, pressing on the nerve inside the ear, reduces hunger. It's acupressure in action. His patients swear it works. Try it. It's safe — if you take care not to get the seed stuck in your ear. And it is certainly not expensive. But since pressure against the nerve is the secret, why couldn't one just use, say, the eraser end of a pencil? — or the rubberized point on the end of a toothbrush handle? Discuss it with your acupuncturist. He or she is sure to have advice.

Back to making your own tape. Your problem may be stress and anxiety. Again, make your own tape. Drink relaxing teas. Michael can be helpful with them. Hanna Kroeger can be helpful. Avoid tranquilizers. Herbal teas and meditation coupled with subliminal tapes can be even more helpful. (See the last chapter for Michael's and Hanna's addresses).

Benign Breast Cysts — Dr. William Ghent, professor of surgery at Queen's University in Kingston, Canada, reports that *diatomic iodine* gave complete pain relief and eliminated cystic lesions in 95% of 700 women to whom he gave the substance. He states that the disease, which is non-malignant, is caused by an iodine deficiency. He states, too, that iodine is essential for normal growth of breast tissue. The patients suffering from fibrocystic problems experience relief within two to eight weeks.

Homeopathic and Other Remedies — Perhaps there is a source near your area from which to purchase your home-opathic supplies. If not, there are several from which you can order. Contact Standard Homeopathic Pharmacy. Or Boer-icke and Tafel. Or Standard Process also offers remedies difficult to purchase elsewhere. Or contact Biological Home-opathic Industries, Inc. Or Boiron-Borneman Homeopathic Products. (See last chapter for addresses.)

National Health Federation and You — The National Health Federation came into existence as a means of repre-senting those of us interested in alternative means of health and healing and in freedom of choice. We (I am a member) have our legislative advocate in Washington D.C., to act as watchguard against legislation detrimental to those of us interested in holistic approaches to healing and medicine. If you are interested in their ongoing struggle on your behalf, in their yearly convention, their list of new age doctors, or in joining in membership, write to the National Health Fed-eration, (address elsewhere). The Federation has long advo-cated "freedom of choice" in health matters and is a strong opponent against those who seek to stop the individual from following the dictates of his or her own conscience in approaches to healing.

Youth and DHEA — Ask at your health store for a tablet called DHEA (dehyroepiandosterone). It contains a compound natural in the body. It's found abundantly in the

bloodstream of the young, but is scarce in the elderly —
which may indicate that its loss contributes to the aging process. Researchers hope DHEA can affect stress hormones.
Stress destroys brain cells responsible for short-term memory,
and adds to the general aging process. So do seek this product
called DHEA.

Memory and Herbs — Concerning memory, Hanna
Kroeger offers an herbal capsule called *Tune In*. She says it
certainly helps to prevent memory loss. She says folks who
use these capsules also report improvement in hearing, which
surprised her. Oh, the wonders of herbs.

DLPA and Pain — Try DL-Phenylalanine (DLPA) as
a pain killer, available at your health store. Taken regularly
it builds up immunity to pain. It's not a drug. It's an amino
acid. Also try Feverfew, an herb, for pain. It's reputed to aid
greatly in migraine headaches. Also at your health store is
a product called Anti-Pain pills, containing buffered aspirin
and DLPA. The combination is extremely effective.

Headaches and Analgesic Oil — For headaches try *White
Flower Analgesic Balm* or *Olbas Oil*. Rubbed on pain spots it's
extremely effective. Try inserting a bit of either oil up each
nostril and inhaling deeply. Also massage your temples and
forehead. Olbas is available from your health store. White
Flower may be ordered from The Trace Co., (address in Chapter 10). Also mix Ben Gay with Tea Tree Oil and massage
on pain area anywhere on the body. It's very effective for
headaches. Avoid applying near eyes.

Magnetic Mattress Pad — To improve your general well-
being, relieve aching joints and muscles, and to even relieve
the pain of arthritis, try sleeping on a *Magnetic Mattress
Pad*. If you can afford one, it is well worth the investment.
I can personally recommend it because I sleep on one. This
mattress pad was uniquely designed by physicians and sci-

entists after many years of research. If you are interested, contact Ruby M. Morrow (address elsewhere).

Liposuction and the Youthful Figure — Liposuction is a means of reduction for hips, waists, abdomens, thighs, arms, necks — anywhere excessive fat has accumulated. It's usually an in-office procedure but may be done in a hospital. Usually it's done with local anesthetics but can be done under general anesthesia. An incision of about one-half inch is made in the selected area and a blunt-ended tubular instrument with an opening near the end is inserted in the incision. A suction unit on the outside end of the instrument draws out the fat by high vacuum pressure. Additional incisions may be necessary to reach various areas. The incisions are closed by sutures, leaving small scars which usually are inconspicuous. There are risks but they seem to be rare: infection and localized collections of blood can be successfully treated. The operation can cause edema — do inquire about it. Also inquire about "lumps" of fat which may remain. Contact your physician or dermatologist for information. The risks in the hands of a skilled surgeon should be minimal.

Youth and Aminoguanidine — Do ask your doctor about a new drug called Aminoguanidine. It's a substance which stimulates action of the body's own cells to wipe out disease, promote inner healing and rejuvenate vital organs. According to Dr. Anthony Cerami, head of the laboratory of medical biochemistry at the Rockefeller University in New York City, this drug "strikes at the cause of aging." Discuss it with your doctor.

Factor X — A team of scientists at the University of Aarhus in Denmark accidentally discovered a natural substance which helps cells keep their vital ability to make life-producing amino acids — which means almost eternal youth. The substance — used as a component in industrial solvents

— is now being tested in laboratories at the University of Nebraska in Omaha. Once the compound passes government safety tests, a face cream will probably be one of the first products created. The compound, called 2-ME, removes wrinkles and reestablishes the youthful elasticity of the skin. Watch for announcements of its release.

Laser Beams — are now being used to eliminate facial wrinkles. The beams are passed over lines and wrinkles much as the check-out girl at the supermarket passes products over the beam. You've been told elsewhere of a doctor already using a similar procedure. See the last chapter for further information.

Live Cell Therapy Cream — A face cream containing sheep cells is now on the market, introduced by heart transplant pioneer, Dr. Christian Barnard. Originally extremely expensive, it now seems to be available at a reduced price. It's called *Glycel*. It can be ordered from Life Essentials (address elsewhere). I've been told, too, that cosmetic surgeons can now inject protein extracted from calf-hide to plump out facial wrinkles. Inquire from your local medical advisory center if interested.

Live Cell Therapy — has long been administered in Europe, especially Switzerland. It's now available in Mexico, just across the border from California — in Tijuana. The therapy is offered by *Genesis West*, a West Germany based biotech company with offices in Redwood City, California. The cells usually are extracted from the organs of the fetuses of sheep. Specific organ extract from the unborn animal vitalizes the same organ in the human into which the extract is injected. The therapy is controversial, but if you're interested, contact Genesis West (address elsewhere). I've already told you elsewhere about their facial rejuvenation process using live cell therapy.

AHA and Natural Alpha Hydroxy Compounds — I've already told you about *New Feeling*, now available at your health store. Its use removes old dead cells that forms the outer layer of your skin, technically called the stratum corneum. This just-released compound "unglues" the excess dead skin cells so that they can be washed away. It's formulated by Durk Pearson and Sandy Shaw, research scientists.

Restored Breast Firmness — The latest word is that cosmetic surgeons are applying electric shock treatments to restore firmness to sagging breasts. The current penetrates and stimulates deep-seated pectoral muscles, making them firm again.

Virility Herbs — You've already read much in previous chapters regarding virility herbs. But there are combinations of others of which you may wish to be aware:

1. Guarana and oat straw;
2. Mexican damiana and licorice leaf;
3. Fenugreek, slippery elm and red clover;
4. Parsley and verbena leaves;
5. Hops, sarsaparilla and basil;
6. Yohimbe bark and mustard seed;
7. Fo-ti-tieng and Korean white ginseng.

Youth Pill — An herbal pill purported to turn back time and rejuvenate the entire being is now available from China. If you're interested, write to The Trace Company for full information.

There you have it! These new plant derivatives may soon be offering eternal youth to the human. We seem to be on the very edge of discovering herbs, extracts and creams that will truly keep the human body forever young.

Chapter Ten

Beauty Products

I promised to tell you more about the products I've recommended and where you might order them.

Fanie International (Therapeutic Skin Treatment Products)

I'll tell you first about Florence and Clyde Johnson and their all-natural products called Fanie (Fan*ay*). The late Clyde Johnson was a formulating chemist for more than a quarter of a century. He dedicated his life to developing and teaching advanced pharmaceutical chemistry as it applies to skin, hair and nails in therapeutic treatments. His work has been recognized and is respected by the medical and cosmetology industry throughout the U.S.A. and internationally for his accomplishments and concepts in the science of skin and chemistry compatibilities.

Florence, a licensed cosmetology instructor, is nationally recognized as a skin care specialist and is endorsed by many national and state associations. As a nationally renowned skin therapist she has worked throughout the nation to establish the importance of medically approved aesthetics. The Fanie line is sold in clinics and salons throughout the United States, Canada, Mexico, Europe and Asia and also under different labels. There are now more than seventy holistic products manufactured by Fanie Laboratories. I've selected only a few to recommend to you.

Of supreme importance is the *White Oak Bark Cleanser* because a radiant healthy skin begins with cleansing. Now what does this brown liquid contain that makes it so remarkable? First, polarized water, which is water with all the impurities removed and to which has been added four-teen different herbs, including: Bermuda kelp, alfalfa, sarsaparilla, black cohosh, saw palmetto, licorice root, sage, mullein, comfrey, fenugreek, hops, cayenne and mint. Plus vitamins and minerals from herbs. Plus PCMX which is an anti fungus, mold inhibitor and full-spectrum bacticide. It prevents oils from becoming rancid. Plus, of course, the white oak bark powder, which is renowned for its healing properties.

Because of its oak bark content, the Cleanser can also be used as a tooth "paste." It heals damaged gums. And as an enema to heal hemorrhoids. And on varicose veins. Just rub it on in the morning and pull your nylons or socks right over it. As a douche it heals vaginal fungus. Just add a teaspoon of the liquid to a quart of warm water. Use the same formula to soak your feet. To heal poison oak, poison ivy, or any other skin blemish, soak in a full tub of warm water to which one tablespoon of Oak Bark Cleanser has been added. It draws out the poisons and impurities. In all these treatments it acts to increase circulation, to be used as a natural poultice to draw out toxins, to heal inflamed areas.

When used as a facial cleansing lotion it need not be followed by an astringent or refreshing lotion, since the white oak bark itself contains a natural anesthetic and astringent. It also automatically contains natural DMSO because it contains the white bark of the oak tree. This amazing product not only thoroughly cleanses but it helps remove dry dead cells.

Fanie's Oak Bark Cleansing Creme — is a white milky liquid which also contains polarized water, hydroprophyl methylcellulose which is seaweed, stearic acid which is the cream base, sweet birch, PCMX and white oak bark.

Both these Cleansers can be followed by any of the Fanie moisturizers. There are too many moisturizers and night creams to be mentioned in detail — they include *Procaine Creme*, *Protein Creme*, *Collagen Creme*, *Apricot Creme*, *Creme D'Orange* for oily skin, *Dreme Creme* for acne skin. They are all natural and contain *no* metals. They are all excellent.

Following the cleansing, spray with the *Misty Mineral Spray* which contains polarized water and a natural astringent, important vitamins and minerals, extracts from herbs and PCMX. It can be used as a refreshing lotion since it also contains mint. You can spray all through the day with this marvelous essence, even over your make-up. Write Karie Hayden or Carlis Orlando, the distributors, for full information.

Fanie's White Oak Shampoo — contains fourteen essential herbs which excel in the treatment of over-permed, damaged, dry, brittle hair. It sloughs off the dead cells of the scalp and feeds the hair shaft. I wouldn't think of using anything else.

Fanie's White Oak Hair Treatment — is a powerful herbal treatment that not only treats the hair and scalp but has been known to prevent baldness and even restore hair. Used once a week the results are often astonishing. The fourteen herbs penetrate the cuticle, the cortex and the medulla of the hair shaft. Because of penetrating natural DMSO, it goes deep into the hair roots to feed them with life force from the herbs. It simultaneously sloughs off dead cells and dissolves oily sebum to allow the bloodstream to reach and feed the roots. The shampoo and Hair Treatment are the same formula, except the Treatment is stronger. The shampoo can be used daily, the Treatment once a week. I discovered these products when my hair went through a thinning stage. I can testify that they have encouraged restoration of my hair. Both shampoo and Treatment are totally natural. No soap, no soap scum, no detergent — nothing but natural ingredients.

Fanie's Sweet Birch Body and Bath Cleanser — This amazing product is excellent to add to a tub bath, only a capful to a tub. It's been known to heal sores and rashes just by soaking in it. It contains polarized water, nettle, the outer layers of deep sea kelp, and sweet birch. It will also help heal itching and inflamed lips of the vagina, and hemorrhoids. For use in the shower just cup your hands for a few drops and splash over your body. Or add a few drops to a bath sponge to aid in removing dead cells all over the body. Add also to infants baths to maintain healthy skin.

Fanie's Body Massage Elastin Lotion — is the ultimate in body cell cleansing and rejuvenation. Whereas most massage lotion contains oils which have long since become rancid, and whereas most oils contain "mother sludge" which harbors bacteria, fungus and mold, Fanie's oils are all fractured to remove such effects, after which the purified oils are stabilized with PCMX to maintain such purification. Fanie's is formulated with a water soluble cream base of polarized water, stearic acid, avocado pulp and oil, vitamins A, C, D, ascorbic acid and essential plant and seed oils. If your massage technician isn't familiar with this product, you may want to enlighten him/her so that you may gain full benefit from your massages.

The Fanie Mask — contains an RNA building block of the cells, so it contains the enzyme lysine. Its deep penetration improves circulation and deposits oxygen and moisture into the deeper levels of the skin. It also contains all twenty-four of the essential amino acids, including stearic acid, glutamic acid, prolene, etc. Also, protein, crude fiber, ash, potassium and PCMX, a natural purifier. It contains absolutely no chemicals. I use it regularly, at least once a week.

Fanie's Tru-Skin — is a mini-mask. It's derived from the outer shell of deep seaweed. It penetrates deeply and helps remove dry dead cells. It's often mixed with the mask powder described above instead of water, to add to the penetrating effect of the "lift-off" of dead cells.

Fanie's Unveil Skin-Peel — As a stronger mini-mask, its prime purpose is to gradually dissolve the very top surface of the skin, slough off dry dead cells, and aid the skin to absorb natural moisturizers. It contains 1% phenol, deep sea kelp, and polarized water. It's the most effective and proven progressive skin peel I have found, except for Fanie's mask — and except for Retinol-A or Retin-A, which requires a doctor's prescription. It can be used daily, resulting in a slight, gentle perpetual skin peel, leaving the skin remarkably free of wrinkles, especially if followed by Fanie's Mist-E-Oil or Fine Line Creme.

Fanie's Mist-E-Oil — is a rich blend of protein oils blended with vitamin E. It's fractured, so it blends with water.

It contains no waxes or paraffins. It should be applied immediately after the mask is removed, to restore the skin's natural oils. Also after cleansing, before moisturizers, at bedtime, or a few drops in your bath water.

Fanie's Fine Line Creme — is a moisturizer. It is especially effective around the eyes and around the mouth where fine lines frequently first begin. It can also be used all over the entire face and throat if you wish. It is formulated from a unique blend of neutral herbal oils, including sesame, sunflower, pumpkin and other seed oils. It also contains cod liver oil which is the highest source of vitamin A. It's also a constrictor which means it tightens the skin. It truly *does*.

Fanie's Herbal Oil — is a rich blend of essential herbal seed oils, containing no waxes or paraffins. Its uses are almost beyond counting. It removes brown spots, moles, warts, some scars, it's even been known to remove skin cancer.

For a personal consultation concerning acne, psoriasis, shingles, wrinkles, dry skin, sun damage, oily skin, excessive facial hair or other problems mentioned; to order any of these products; or for further information concerning any of the Fanie Products, write to: Karie Hayden or Carlis Orlando, 975 Hornblend #D, San Diego, CA 92109 or P.O. Box 81502, San Diego, CA 92138. Or call them at (619)581-3321.

Or contact Valjean McGinty, Oma Enterprises, P.O. Box 4873, Palm Springs, CA 92264 to order Fanie Products. Or you can write to Florence Johnson at 1645 Reynolds Ave., Irvine, CA 92714 or call 1-800-441-FANI to get the name of the Fanie representative in your area.

Creative Illusion Cosmetics

Karie Hayden and Carlis Orlando have just created an incredible line of cosmetics that sell under the brand name of *Creative Illusion*. Both of these esthetician-educators have given years of their lives toward creating and marketing cosmetics as pure as can be found anywhere. These cosmetics have only now become available. Their lipsticks contain castor oil, candelilla wax (from the candelilla plant), and propylparben BHA (a fungus inhibitor). The foundation contains isocetyl stearate, caccarilla bark, koalin (China clay), stearic acid (vegetable oil), isoprople-lanolate for pigmentation and methylparaben, a preservative. They offer a full selection of cosmetics — make-up foundation, cake blushes, eyebrow and eyeliners, lipsticks, powder, mascara — all formulated as near "natural" as anywhere available. Their foundation is oil free and is superb! — their lipsticks beautiful — and their mascara even stimulates the growth of sparse eyelashes. It contains candelilla wax from plants and orokerit, a natural mineral. Do contact them for full information and order form. Again: 975 Hornblend, Suite D, San Diego, CA 92109. Telephone (619)581-3321.

Beleza Beauty Creams

The next brand of skin products I can heartily endorse is called *Beleza* (Bel-et-za) *Beauty Cream*. Beleza is unique and entirely different from any other cream known in Europe or America. The original Italian formula was created years ago by a distinguished scientist, a member of the Di Mascatelli family in Milano, Italy. Its original purpose was for use by the medical profession to aid in the treatment of severe skin conditions, but it came to be recognized as a means of restoring youthful skin. It is completely natural. It contains penetrating herbs to achieve the proper subcutaneous stimulation and circulation so necessary for retaining a youthful wrinkle-free skin.

The anti-aging formula, which I use constantly, contains pure raw honey, which acts as a powerful nondrying astringent and peel. Its sea kelp gives it antiseptic qualities. Its herbs heal and restore firmness. It contains vitamins A, E and D, plus B1, B2, B6, and B12 to gently slough off dead cells and dry scaly skin. Its astonishing formula results in an excellent moisturizer. It contains all 22 amino acids and 56 vitamins and minerals in all. It contains a collagen complex plus calcium to restore elastin and natural collagen. Its anti-aging ingredients heal rashes, burns and scar tissues. It contains essential nucleic acids (RNA-DNA) to stimulate new cell growth. Beleza also offers a formula for acne, one for cleansing, and an excellent facial mask.

I constantly use Beleza Anti-Aging Formula as a night cream, and have for years. I use it to perform my facial massage when I waken, using upward strokes as described by Sanford Bennett. You wouldn't believe the results! — the removal of dead cells and the resulting freshness. I can enthusiastically endorse *all* the Beleza products. Direct any inquiries for further information to Sandra Joan, The Sanfy Corp., 850 N. Cypress St., Orange, CA 92667.

Patricia Allison Products

Many years ago when I was seeking natural products for my make-up, I met Patricia Allison, who was totally involved in creating such a line. Patti, during the '50s, was concerned with the biological compatibility of the then-available skin and hair care products. One by one, she developed products blending the best of nature and science to provide natural beauty enhancement even for hypersensitive and problem skins. This line has continued to evolve over the last thirty years, and is being continuously tested on all types of human skin and scalps. Her company has been awarded the honored Beauty Without Cruelty Seal of Approval for *not* testing her products on animals. Additionally, the skin and hair care formulas contain no added color; most are available without fragrance; and most contain no animal ingredients. Where used, animal ingredients are limited to lanolin (derived from wool), honey, and beeswax.

Patti has now retired from the daily business regimen. Although Ann and Tom Keenan now own the company, Patti is still actively involved as a consultant and product tester. I am particularly anxious to make you aware of the Allison cosmetics — the make-up base, rouge, lipstick, and powder which are as natural as any available. I can certainly endorse their excellence. Although I use *Fanie Cleansing Formula*, I often use Patricia's *Vita Balm* as a moisturizer under make-up. One of the highlights of the line, *Vita Balm* was originally created with a doctor's guidance for burn therapy — but they discovered its deep-moisturizing proteins imparted resilience, smoothness, and firmness to the skin. Also, it was found to bring normalcy to men's hands after exposure to auto repair, cement work, gardening, etc.

I can't add much to what I've already told you about her *Wild Fern Freshener*, except that it is formulated from an herbal infusion, aqueous vitamin E, and essential oils.

Also it contains no fermented alcohols or aluminum derivatives. I've told you, too, about her sunscreen, her *Babyskin Masque*, her *Swedish Scrub*. She offers many other products but her cosmetics are the products I'm most familiar with. Her foundations are excellent. She offers a white undercoat to cover lines and wrinkles, or to mix with other shades to create a shade of your choice. Her cake blush, applied with a brush, doesn't "blotch" as do some powdered blushes. She offers hard-to-find pink lipsticks. To contact her, direct inquiries to: Patricia Allison, 4470 Monahan Road, La Mesa, CA 92041.

HANNA KROEGER— is known worldwide. She distributes her remedies, mostly herbal and homeopathic, to a vast clientele. Though she has more interest in health than in you
th and beauty, I have included her in this book because who cares about youth or beauty if one isn't healthy. You can read fully about her and her remedies in *The You Book: A Treasury of Health and Healing*. Hanna has received many of her formulas through inspiration and guidance from Higher Sources. She is a walking encyclopedia for health restoration and maintenance. Whatever your problem, whether health, youth or beauty, write to her at 1122 Pearl Street, Boulder, CO 80302. Her phone number is (303)443-0261.

LESLEY and **MICHAEL TIERRA**— know as much about herbal science as anyone I know. They present seminars throughout the world. If you have a health problem, they have an herbal remedy. They also have herbal rejuvenation remedies. Write them for literature at: P.O. Box 712, Santa Cruz, CA 95061.

Other Recommended Products and People

Abdominizer: Abdominizer, 6 Fitness Quest Plaza, Canton, OH 44750.

Acupuncture and Facelift: Master Sehan Kim, 3875 Wilshire Blvd., #704, Los Angeles, CA 90010; (213)462-6795.

Air Ionizing Wave: Hair by Nelda, 158-A W. Foothill Blvd., Upland, CA 91786; (714)920-0333 If no answer, call (714) 985-6244.

Bar Magnet: Bio Health Enterprises, Inc. Rt.3, Box 121, Murray, KY 42071.

Edgar Cayce Products: Cayce Corner, 4018 N. 40th St., Phoenix, AZ 85018; (602)955-0551.

Date Sugar: Shields Date Gardens, Indio, CA 92201.

Deodorant Crystals: B&K Products, 5083 Camelot Dr., Mobile, AL 36619.

Face Peel: Dr. Robert Harmon, Desert Medical Center, 43-576 Washington St., Bermuda Dunes, CA 92201; (619)345-2696.

G+: Dynapro International, P.O. Box 3002, Ogden, UT 84409.

GH3 (Gerovital): Valjean McGinty, Oma Enterprises, P.O. Box 4873, Palm Springs, CA 92264.

Glycel Live Cell Therapy Cream: Life Essentials, 8306 Wilshire Blvd., #550, Beverly Hills, CA 90211

Hair Brush: Hoffritz, 515 W. 24th St., New York, NY 10011-1182.

Laser Resurfacing: Dr. Lawrence David, Hermosa Skin Medical Clinic, 415 Pier Ave., Hermosa Beach, CA 90254.

Live Cell Therapy Cream: Swanson Health Product, P.O. Box 2803, Fargo, ND 58108; (800)437-4148.

Live Cell Therapy: Genesis West, 241 Hazel Ave. Dept. 3, Redwood City, CA 94061 or Call Toll Free: (800)227-8823. California residents call collect: (415)365-6692.

Ma Evans Herbal Hair Lotion : E.P.I. Inc., P.O. Box 719, Dunedin, FL 33528.

Magnetic Mattress Pad: Ruby M. Morrow, 10210 Baseline Rd. Sp. 238, Alta Loma, CA 91701; (714)-944-3708.

Mineral Salt: The Dews Co., P.O. Box 147, Mineral Wells, TX 76067.

Mixed seeds, goat's milk whey, yeast flakes and other products: Arthur Blackmer, National Fruit and Vegetable Industries, P.O.Box 92643, Pasadena, CA 91109.

National Health Federation: P.O. Box 688, Monrovia, CA 91016.

New Feeling and other Life Extension Products: P.O. Box 8190, Santa Cruz, CA 95061.

Novadermy: Vitachem Int. Inc., 241 Hazel Ave., Redwood City, CA 94061. Call Toll Free: (800)227-8823. California residents call collect: (415)365-6692.

Oriental Pearl Cream: 6835 Valjean Ave., Van Nuys, CA 91406; (818)785-0952.

Pillow, Chiropractic Special Contoured: Dr. Noll Walker, P.O. Box 2052, Upland, CA 91785-2052.

Real Salt: American Orsa, Inc., 75 N. State, Redmund, UT 84652; (801)529-7487.

Retinol-A: Fanie Products (Address given in beginning of chapter.)   (or)

E. Burnham Co. 4560 W. Touhy Ave. Dept. WW228, Lincolnwood, IL 60646.

Silken Earth: Aubrey Organics, Tampa, Florida 33614. Available at health stores.

Small Pillow: Solutions, Box 6878, Dept. SLSC 88, Portland, OR 97228.

Sul-Ray Acne Treatment Cream: Alvin Last, Inc, Dobbs Ferry, NY 10522.

Sunrider Products: Dr. Noll Walker (See address under "Pillow").

Swanson Health Products: P.O. Box 2803, Fargo, ND 58108; (800)437-4148.

Travel Pillow; Wrinkle-Reducing Pillow;Facial Sauna; Humidifier; Whirlpool Bathtub Spa: Hammacher Schlemmer, Midwest Operations Center, 11013 Kenwood Rd., Cincinnati, OH 45242.

White Flower Analgesic Balm: The Trace Co., Box 6050, Beverly Hills, CA 90212.

Homeopathic Remedies:

Dr. Edward Bach Center, Mt. Vernon, Sotwell Wallingford, Oxon, OX10, OPZ, England.

Boericke and Tafel, 1011 Arch St., Philadelphia, PA 19107; (215)922-2967.

Boiron-Borneman Homeopathic, 1208 Amosland Rd., Box 54, Norwood,PA 19074; (215)532-2035.

Herbal Home Products, Box 258, Rescue, CA 95672; (916)626-5046.

Similia Laboratories, Inc., 5946 Okeechobee Blvd., West Palm Beach, FL 33417.

Standard Homeopathic Pharmacy, Box 61067, Los Angeles, CA 90061.

Standard Process, 2401 South Atlantic Blvd., Commerce, CA 90040; (800)372-7218.

Biological Homeopathic, 11600 Cochiti S.E., Albuquerque, NM 87123.